A STRAIGHT TALKING INTRODUCTION TO

EMOTIONAL WELLBEING

FROM MENTAL ILLNESS TO MAD STUDIES

A revised second edition of
A Straight Talking Introduction to Being a Mental Health Service User

PETER BERESFORD

PCCS BOOKS

First published 2010 as *A Straight Talking Introduction to Being a Mental Health Service User*

This edition published 2023

PCCS Books Ltd
Wyastone Business Park
Wyastone Leys
Monmouth
NP25 3SR
UK

Tel +44 (0)1600 891509
contact@pccs-books.co.uk
www.pccs-books.co.uk

A Straight Talking Introduction to Emotional Wellbeing: From mental illness to Mad Studies

British Library Cataloguing in Publication Data.
A catalogue record for this book is available from the British Library

ISBNs
paperback – 978 1 915220 35 6
epub – 978 1 915220 36 3

Cover design by Jason Anscomb
Printed in the UK by Severnprint, Gloucester

Praise for *A Straight Talking Introduction to Emotional Wellbeing: From mental illness to Mad Studies*

This book represents a mission, a historical analysis of the radical challenges in mental health and social care to address a truly equitable, lived and experienced epistemological framework. One that liberates those who have been misdiagnosed, criminalised and endured death. It transcends race and equality and offers the potential for equity from assessment, admission, care planning and discharge, beyond the restraints of a new slavery in the neoliberal economics of modern mental health care. It empowers black men like me, the victims of a new drapetomania, to seek clinical parity, to use my values as capital in exchange for a move away from the biomedical entrapment to a caring mental health system built on the values of liberation and humanity. The book offers a reform beyond principles of care and autonomy. It legislates for a coproduction based on the erosion of professionalised medical dominance and the recognition of the service user as the advocate of political and statutory change in mental health care.
Colin King, Black survivor research activist and founder of the Whiteness and Race Equality Network

Peter Beresford takes us on a journey though the ideas, values and actions of service users, survivors and disabled people, mapping his own steps on the way. He speaks with clarity, never obscuring with academic language the important ideas he discusses. This is a compelling critique and a hopeful vision, proposing ways in which we can address the seemingly intractable problems with how madness and distress are conceived and treated. At a time of crisis in mental health, this book is energising and encouraging.
Dr Sarah Carr, independent researcher and Visiting Senior Research Fellow, Service User Research Enterprise, Institute of Psychiatry, Psychology and Neuroscience, King's College London

Whether you're a healthcare provider, a researcher or someone who uses services, this book is helpful to anybody who wants to learn more about the many facets of mental health care and treatments. The book demonstrates the value of service users' voices by including points of view that remind us of the importance of first-person experiential knowledge in contributing to the radical changes needed to improve public policy, law and healthcare itself. The book also takes readers a step further by discussing the exciting theoretical possibilities available through the work of Mad Studies and its role in addressing and moving us all closer to a collective politics of hope and survival.

Lucy Costa, Deputy Executive Director, The Empowerment Council

With incisiveness and depth, Peter Beresford presents a comprehensive picture of the mental 'help' system as it currently operates, which is largely to deepen suffering, prejudice and isolation. Interweaving the personal with peer narratives, he offers hope in the liberatory potential of user/survivor alliances, as opposed to individual helplessness and bleakness engendered by mainstream treatments. This is a book that saddens in parts, yet also drives in the meaningfulness of organising together and becoming agents of our own lives and stories, instead of passive consumers within a heartless, indifferent machine that effaces the person and sees them only as a social nuisance to be kept in control. This is a book I recommend to everyone who believes psychiatry has a solution for them and that, sooner or later, they are going to heal using those unending, ever-increasing pharmacological prescriptions.

Prateeksha Sharma, peer psychotherapist and author of *Barriers to Recovery from 'Psychosis': A peer investigation of psychiatric subjectivation*

A Straight Talking Introduction to Emotional Wellbeing: From mental illness to Mad Studies

Contents

Dedications

This book is dedicated to all the mental health service users/survivors I have met on my own journey through the system and through service user organisations, who are no longer with us. People like me owe them a lot. It is also dedicated to those still making or who have yet to make that journey, wishing them my best and every support possible.

Since this book was first published, three pioneering mental health service user/survivor activists key to its writing have died. They are Peter Campbell, Patricia Chambers and Jan Wallcraft. This second edition is dedicated to them and their memory, and to all the other survivors who have died too soon and been lost to us. We all owe them so much.

About the author

Peter Beresford OBE is a long-term user of mental health services and Co-Chair of Shaping Our Lives, the national independent service user-controlled organisation and network. He is also Visiting Professor at the University of East Anglia, Emeritus Professor of Citizen Participation at Essex University and Emeritus Professor of Social Policy and Director of the Centre for Citizen Participation at Brunel University. He has a longstanding involvement in issues of participation and empowerment as a writer, researcher, educator, service user and campaigner. He is co-editor, with Jasna Russo, of the *Routledge International Handbook of Mad Studies* (2022).

About the series editors

Richard Bentall is Professor of Clinical Psychology at the University of Sheffield and has previously held chairs at Liverpool, Manchester, and Bangor universities. He is a Fellow of the British Psychological Society and of the British Academy. His research has focused on the cognitive and emotional mechanisms involved in psychotic symptoms such as hallucinations and delusions, and also examined why social risk factors (for example childhood adversities) provoke the cognitive and emotional changes that lead to these symptoms. He has also conducted clinical trials of novel psychological treatments for psychosis.

Pete Sanders was a counsellor, educator, clinical supervisor and author for more than 30 years, and co-founder of PCCS Books. He wrote numerous articles on psychotherapy and mental health, and several books, including *First Steps in Counselling* (now in its 5th edition (PCCS Books, 2022) and *The Person-Centred Counselling Primer* (PCCS Books, 2006). Pete died in February 2022.

Acknowledgements

There are many people to thank for their help in writing this book and its second edition. First, the group of mental health service users/survivors who came together to help inform the book through their discussion and whose collective words I have quoted: Lucia Franco, Adrian Tibbs, Colin Dean and John Clark. Then the survivors who I have quoted individually in the book, who were all kind enough to put down their views for me to include. I'd also like to thank Wendy Bryant, formerly of Brunel University London and now the University of Essex; the late Pete Sanders from PCCS Books, for his patience and encouragement (that may not be strong enough a word!); Catherine Jackson and the team at PCCS Books for their continuing support, and especially Sandy Green for her sensitive editing of the first edition, which greatly improved the book. Also, my friends and colleagues, survivors Louise Pembroke and Peter Campbell (who is sadly no longer with us) for the longstanding understanding and inspiration I have gained from them. Also, the Survivors' History Group and electronic website for the constant insights I have gained from them. My thanks also to Simon Kewer for his illustrations for the book and the late Jan Wallcraft for her foreword. She lives on through her wise words,

One of the things I did when I knew I was going to write an updated version of this book was to tweet about it and ask survivors on radical survivor websites and Facebook group sites, like Drop the Disorder! and the Mad Studies Group, what they thought I should include in it. I got lots of helpful suggestions. A key one was that the discussion needed to be put in an international context and that any proposals for reform should challenge, not perpetuate, existing inequalities at every level, from personal to global. In this age of globalisation and internationally entrenched neoliberal ideology, comments also highlighted the importance of addressing the issues facing indigenous peoples and peoples of the Global South. They also highlighted issues of addressing diversity and exploring identity politics. I have tried to do this and want to thank everyone who responded and helped in this process.

Most of all of course I would like to thank the many people who have given me support, kept me going and helped me to gain understanding through my experience of madness and distress and the mental health system and all those who have helped make the survivor and Mad Studies movements what they are and can be.

Thank you.

Introducing the *Straight Talking Introductions* series

What are mental health problems?

Much of what is written and spoken about emotional distress or mental health problems implies that they are illnesses. This can lead us all too easily to believe that we no longer have to think about mental health problems, because illness is best left to doctors. They are the illness experts, and psychiatrists are the doctors who specialise in mental illness. This series of books is different because we don't think that all mental health problems should automatically be regarded as illnesses.

If mental health problems aren't necessarily illnesses, it means that the burden of responsibility for distress in our lives should not be shouldered entirely by doctors and psychiatrists. All citizens have a responsibility, however small, in creating a world where everyone has a decent opportunity to live a fulfilling life. This is a contentious idea, but one that we want to advance, alongside the dominant medical view.

Rather than accept that the ways of understanding and solutions to mental health problems are 'owned' by the medical profession, we will take a good look at alternatives that involve the users of psychiatric services, their carers, families, friends and other 'ordinary people' taking control of their own lives, and that means all of us. One of the tools required in order to become active in mental health issues, whether your own or other people's, is knowledge. This series of books is a starting point for anyone who wants to know more about mental health.

How these books are written

Information

We want these books to be understandable, so we use everyday language wherever possible. The books could have been almost completely jargon-free, but we thought that including some technical and medical terms would be helpful. Most doctors, psychiatrists and psychologists use the medical model of mental illness and manuals to help them diagnose mental health problems. The medical model and the diagnostic manuals use a particular set of terms to describe what doctors think of as 'conditions'. Although these words aren't very good at describing individual people's experiences, they are used a lot in psychiatric and psychological services, so we thought it would be helpful to define these terms as we went along and use them in a way that might help readers understand what the professionals mean. We don't expect that psychiatrists and psychologists and others working in mental health services will stop using medical terminology (although we think it would be respectful for them to drop it when talking to their patients and their families), so these books should help you get used to and learn *their* language.

The books also contain resources for further learning. As well as lists of books, websites and organisations at the end of the book, there are references. These will not be important to everyone, but they do tell the reader where information – a claim about effectiveness, an argument for or against, or a quotation – has come from, so you can follow it up if you wish.

Being realistic and reassuring

Our aim is to be realistic – neither overly optimistic nor pessimistic. Things are nearly always more complicated than we would like them to be. Honest evaluations of mental health problems, of what might cause them, of what can help and of what the likely outcome might be are, like so much in life, somewhere in between. For the vast majority of people, it would be wrong to say that they have an illness from which they will never recover. But it would be equally wrong to say that they will be completely unchanged by the distressing thoughts and feelings they are having. Life is an accumulation of experiences. There is almost certainly no pill, or any other treatment for that matter, that will take us back to 'how we were before'. There are many things we can do (and we look at lots of them in this series), in collaboration with doctors, psychiatrists, psychologists and counsellors, and, indeed, everyone working in mental health services, with the help of our friends and family, or on our own, that stand a good chance of helping us feel better and build a constructive life, with hope for the future.

Of course, we understand that the experiences dealt with in these books can sometimes be so overwhelming, confusing and terrifying that people will try to escape from them by withdrawing, going mad or even trying to kill themselves. This happens when our usual coping strategies fail us. We accept that killing oneself is, in some circumstances, a rational act – that, for the person in question, it can make a lot of sense. Nonetheless, we believe that much of the distress that underpins such an extreme course of action, from which there can be no turning back, is avoidable. For this reason, all of the books in this series point towards realistic hope and recovery.

Debates

There is no single convenient answer to many of the most important questions explored in these books. No matter how badly we might wish for a simple answer, what we have is a series of debates – or arguments, more like – between stakeholders, and there are many stakeholders whose voices demand space in these books. We use the word 'stakeholders' here because service users, carers, friends, family, doctors, psychologists, psychiatrists, nurses and other healthcare workers, scientists in drug companies, therapists and, indeed, all citizens have a stake in how our society understands and deals with problems of mental health. It is simultaneously big business and intimately personal, and many things in between. As we go along, we try to explain how someone's stake in distress (including our own, where we can see it), whether professional or personal, can influence their experience and judgement.

While we want to present competing (sometimes opposing) viewpoints, we don't want to leave the reader high and dry to evaluate complicated debates on their own. We will try to present reasonable conclusions that might point in certain directions for personal action. Above all, though, we believe that knowledge is power and that the better informed you are, even though the information might be conflicting, the more able you will be to make sound decisions.

It's also useful to be reminded that the professionals involved in helping distressed people are themselves caught in the same flow of conflicting information. It is their *job*, however, to interpret it in our service, so that the best solutions are available to as many people as possible. You may have noticed that the word 'best' brings with it certain challenges, not least defining what we mean when we use this term. Perhaps 'the best' means the most effective? However, even using words like 'effective' doesn't completely clear up the puzzle. An effective treatment for an employer could be the one that returns a member of staff to work quickly; for a parent, it could be one that makes their child feel happier and calmer. For the government or the NHS, or someone running a private healthcare business, 'effective' might mean 'cost-effective'. This brings us to evidence.

Evidence

Throughout these books there will be material that we will present as 'evidence'. This is one of the most contentious terms to be found in this series. One person's evidence is another person's fanciful mythology and yet another person's oppressive propaganda. Nevertheless, the term crops up increasingly in everyday settings, most relevantly when we hear of 'evidence-based practice'. The idea behind this term is that the treatments psychologists and psychiatrists offer should be those that 'work'. Crudely put, there should be some evidence that, say, talking about problems or taking a prescribed drug actually helps people feel better. We encounter a real problem, however, when trying to evaluate this evidence, as the books in this series will demonstrate. We will try not to discount any 'evidence' out of hand, but we will critically evaluate it, and we will do this with a bias towards scientific evaluation.

The types of evidence that will be covered in these books, along with their positive and negative points, include the following.

Research methods, numbers and statistics

On the one hand, the logic of most research is simple, but on the other hand, the way things have to be arranged to avoid bias in the results can lead to a perplexing system of measurements. Even the experts lose the sense of it, sometimes. We'll try to explain the logic of studies, but almost certainly leave out the details. You can look these up yourself if you wish.

The books in this series look at research into a wide range of issues relating to mental health problems, including the experience of distress, what is known about the causes of problems, and their prevention and treatment. Different research methods are appropriate for each of these areas, so we will be looking at different types of research as we go along. We say this now because many readers may be most familiar with studies into the *effective treatments* of distress, and we want to emphasise that there are many other credible and valid sources of essential information about distress that are sometimes overlooked.

You may have come across the idea that some research methods are 'better' than others – that they constitute a 'gold standard'. In the case of research into the effectiveness of different treatments, the gold standard is usually considered to be randomised controlled trials (RCTs). In simple terms, RCTs are complex (and often very expensive) experiments in which a group of individuals who all suffer from the same problem are allocated randomly to a treatment (such as a drug or a form of talking therapy) or a 'control' treatment (at its simplest, no treatment at all, or a dummy pill or 'placebo') to test if the treatment works. We are not necessarily convinced that RCTs always *are* the best way of proving the effectiveness of different treatments, but they are, currently, the method given most credence by the bodies that control funding and what it is spent on, such as (in England) the National Institute for Health and Care Excellence (NICE) – so we need to understand them.

Before it is accepted by academics and clinicians, research must be written up and published in a journal that asks independent people to read it, to make sure that it is *bona fide* and that no glaring mistakes have been made. In recent years, a number of high-profile academics and scientific commentators have drawn attention to possible problems with this system of quality control. This series of books is not the place to deal with these arguments, but where they impinge on the evidence in a particular area, we will make sure it is highlighted.

Personal experience

Personal experience is an important source of evidence, to the extent that, nowadays, people who have suffered debilitating psychiatric distress are sometimes called 'experts by experience'. Personal stories provide an essential counterbalance to the impersonal numbers and statistics often found in research projects such as RCTs. While not everyone is average, by definition most people are. Balancing the average results obtained from RCTs with some personal stories helps complete the picture and is now widely accepted, to the extent that it has given birth to the new field of 'survivor research'.

Understanding contexts

Widening our view to include people's families and lives and the cultural, economic, social and political settings in which we live completes the picture. Mental health problems are connected to the conditions in which we all live, just as much as they are connected to our biology. From the start, we want readers to know that, if there is one message or model that these books are trying to get across, it is that problems in mental health are more often than not the result of complex events in the environments in which we live and our reactions to them. These reactions can also be influenced by our biology and the way we have learned to think and feel. Hopefully, these books will help disentangle the puzzle of distress and provide positive suggestions and hope for us all, whether we work in the system, currently have mental health problems ourselves or are caring for or friends with someone who has.

We hope that readers of these books will feel empowered by what they learn and thereby feel more able to get the best out of mental health services. It would be wonderful if our efforts, directly or indirectly, influence the development of services that effectively address the emotional, social and practical needs of people with mental health problems.

Richard Bentall
Pete Sanders
2021

Foreword to the first edition
Jan Wallcraft

Peter Beresford has been an inspiration to me and to many other service users/survivors as we try to make sense of our lives in this 'maddening' world, as Peter terms it in his Postscript.

All Peter's work and writing is done openly as someone who has experienced mental distress and psychiatric treatment. He works consistently to challenge medical assumptions about mental distress and psychiatric labelling and to help people to take power over their own lives.

Peter is never afraid to be controversial but does not make cheap points to get headlines. He always ensures that his work is based on the lived experience of mental health service users and disabled people. He writes in language that is free from jargon and clearly sets out the views of a wide range of people who have been on the receiving end of state services.

Many of us have reason to be thankful for the articles he has written in the *Guardian*, his dedicated work to involve service users and carers in social work policy and education, and his commitment to supporting service user-led research.

Straight talking is indeed needed; so is the openness and courage that Peter himself models in his work.

This book is timely, coming at a point in history [it was first published in 2010] when a new government is intent on changing the landscape of mental health and social services yet again, with renewed attacks on so-called 'benefits scroungers' and those with long-term needs for services and support.

This book is based on Peter's interviews with service users, and a wide range of research evidence.

As is pointed out throughout this book, it is not rare to have mental health problems or to be a friend or family member of someone who does, yet mental health problems are still widely misunderstood, resulting in those who have a problem with their mental health being afraid to ask for help. Many of those who receive treatment do not find it helpful, and many end up feeling excluded because of the attitudes of others.

The book guides the reader through the 'parallel universe' of the mental health system and explains the mental health service user/survivor movement set up to challenge our exclusion from the mainstream. It explores issues for a range of minority groups who often face even worse discrimination and exclusion.

It looks at how service users share support and information, advocate for one another, get involved in trying to change the system and create alternatives. It explores how social models of disability and mental health are posing a fundamental challenge to exclusion by developing concepts such as independent living with ongoing support as needed.

Finally, Peter sets out a vision for the future, acknowledging that it is not just the psychiatric system, but the world that needs changing. He sets out key principles for change that can be achieved if we work together, as individuals taking back our own power and through our networks and alliances.

This book offers valuable information, a message of hope and a call for collective action for real, sustainable change through practical strategies such as rights-based, anti-oppressive practice, support for independent living, building the capacity of service user groups and enabling service user-led research and services. I wish it had been available when I was beginning my own recovery from mental distress and psychiatric treatment, and I hope it is widely read and shared by mental health service users and survivors and those who care for or about them.

Dr Jan Wallcraft
Survivor researcher; Honorary Fellow, University of Birmingham; Visiting Fellow, University of Hertfordshire

Introduction to the second edition

It's now 13 years since the first edition of this book was published, in 2010. What's interesting is what has and hasn't happened since then. UK mental health services were in crisis then. The situation has gone from bad to worse since, and often the talk is of permanent crisis.

This probably reached its worst-ever point early in 2023. An investigation into NHS mental health services in Essex – thought to be the largest in the UK – came under public pressure to be upgraded to a full public inquiry. The probe into the deaths of 2000 people in the county over 20 years had 'stalled', and the then Health Secretary was reported to favour an upgrade into a full public enquiry that would compel current and former medics to give evidence (Campbell, 2022; Gallagher, 2023).

This reflects a deteriorating national situation with no improvement on the horizon. More generally, resourcing is even more inadequate, and mental health service users and those in difficulties even worse served. The situation internationally is really no better, with enormous resources committed to a so-called global mental health policy that seeks to extend and impose psychiatry even beyond its existing wide borders, regardless of the widespread current questioning of it, its evident inadequacy and its colonialistic tendencies.

The establishment mantra that mental health is the same as physical health rings less and less true. This is not only because of the differences in resourcing and attitudes towards the mental and physical health sectors, but also because of an experiential narrative growing in power that this just isn't so. There aren't many physical illnesses that leave people stigmatised, isolated and feared in the ways that the 'mental illness' label does.

However, it is this challenging of old understandings of madness and distress where we can see change. Of course, it's been a rocky ride. Efforts to involve mental health service users/survivors, and for us to be involved, have faced at least as many barriers as encouragements. Efforts to tokenise and incorporate people's aims and actions are, if anything, even more concerted. Yet, very important positive things have also been happening. The genie of survivor involvement really has been let out of the bottle and it is difficult to see how it will ever be forced back. No less important, a whole coherent discipline – or, as some have called it, 'indiscipline' – has emerged. This is the praxis of Mad Studies. Its significance is that it is a concerted movement for both action and intellectual change. This is what past survivor struggles have often lacked and, in my opinion at least, by offering a cohesive basis for thought and collective change, it massively ups the challenge to the individualising and medicalising of 'mental health'. This and other key developments, such as the new emphasis on experiential knowledge, decolonisation, white privilege and the emergence of the #MeToo and Black Lives Matter movements, have all created new space, new energy and new ideas to help any of us experiencing madness and distress or using mental health services. So yes, many things have got worse, but counter-pressures give us hope.

At the same time, there can be little doubt that the world is an even more uncertain place than it was when this book was first published. Threats to the planet have grown rather than abated, and commitments to challenge them have, if anything, been further diluted. The evidence for the destructive impacts of climate change has increased beyond question. Global problems of poverty, inequality, ill health and early death have grown rather than been reduced. International conflict has worsened and, as I write, has extending again to the European mainland in the grim war between the Ukraine and Russia.

All of these have inevitably been associated with increasingly destructive consequences at a personal level, creating more uncertainty, insecurity, conflict and difficulties for more and more of us. And one of the expressions of such damage is the pressures placed on our mental as well as physical wellbeing.

That is the focus of this book, where we try to make sense of the problems facing us and turn particularly to the insights, understanding and experience of those living with those problems to work out how to achieve better lives and a better world for the future for all of us.

Introduction to the first edition

> I believe in the need to generate knowledge from the perspective of the least powerful groups in society. Within mental health research, this means discovery and exploration with and for the people who use and refuse psychiatric services.
> *Angela Sweeney (2009)*

The aim of this book is to talk clearly and openly about an issue that is highly contentious and that raises strong emotions, particularly fear. There is no agreed terminology in this field; instead, there is talk of mental health problems, madness, mental illness and distress, as well as the routine use of many demeaning terms like 'nutter' and 'loony'. This is a book about making sense of being a mental health service user. It is an issue in which many people and groups have an interest: policymakers, politicians, economists, professionals, family, friends and loved ones and, of course, service users themselves. Thus, interest may arise for occupational, political, financial, academic or personal reasons – or any combination of the above. The reasons people directly experiencing madness and distress have for such interest – people now increasingly called 'service users' or 'survivors', as many like to be called – are the most direct and can be expected to be the most intense. It is a generally negative identity that dominates and damages our lives. Historically, it is also one that has been among the most devalued and least documented. Yet mental health service users have unique experience, knowledge and understandings to offer. That is why this book not only focuses on being a mental health service user but is also written by and from the perspective of someone who has used mental health services long term.

Interest in the perspectives of mental health service users/ survivors reflects a broader policy and political interest in the views and experience of people on the receiving end of policy and politics. In recent years in the UK and internationally, there has been a new interest in 'user-centred' and 'user-led' practice and provision in many areas of policy, from education and health to housing and leisure. There has been an official interest in involving service users, consulting with them and listening to their views. We will look more at the reasons for this later. But this raises some particular issues in relation to mental health services and mental health service users that need to be considered carefully. This is because mental health policy can and does restrict people's rights, as well as being intended to provide support. Mental health service users are still frequently seen as threatening and dangerous, as well as in need of help. This raises questions about how we can make involvement and user-led services real for this group and how they can influence what happens to them when, in reality, in some cases, restrictions are imposed on their human and civil rights and on the control they have over their own lives.

It is not only that service users/survivors may have a particular previously neglected perspective to offer. We/they also have important new insights to contribute about 'mental health', madness, distress and the responses made to them. Since the 1960s, big challenges have emerged to psychiatry and traditional understandings of 'mental health' and 'mental illness'. But initially these mainly came from within psychiatry and related professions themselves: from radical psychiatric thinkers and clinicians like Thomas Szasz, the anti-psychiatrists of the 1960s and 1970s – notably R.D. Laing – and critical psychologists and psychiatrists and radical social workers.

More recently, from the 1980s, new critiques began to emerge from service users/survivors themselves. These have much to tell us both about being a mental health service user and about the services and systems that define us. Even more important, perhaps, they point to new ways of understanding and addressing madness and distress. That is why this book in the series has a contribution to make not only in terms of telling us more about service users and their understandings of themselves and the world they inhabit, but also in making clear what perpetuates madness and distress, how such phenomena and experiences may best be understood and prevented, and how people can be best supported to deal with them as successfully as possible.

This book draws on many people's experiences, ideas and proposals. These are mainly but not exclusively people with first-hand experience of mental distress and of using mental health services. I have also learned from professionals and practitioners in the field, and educators and researchers – and sometimes these have been people who also have direct experience of using mental health services, although this may not be something they feel able to talk about. These are people I have got to know and worked with, and whose writings and discussions I have learned from. I have also had discussions with some mental health service users specifically as part of writing this book, so it can be informed by their knowledge, experience and understandings.

The aim of this book is to help us make better sense of our and other people's experience as mental health service users and also to be able to play a more active role in society, individually and collectively, by building on the strengths of that experience.

I should say that, when this happened to me and I felt I was going mad, I was in every sense in a state of confusion, panic and disorientation. I didn't understand what was happening. I didn't really know where to turn to. I wasn't really able to act in the calm and thoughtful way most helpful to sorting out any problem or emergency. Those around me were probably little better equipped. That's when I could really have benefitted from the kind of experiential knowledge I have tried to put together here.

The structure of the book

Chapter 1 sets the scene, introducing the author and considering the experience of being a mental health service user/survivor. Chapter 2 offers a broad view of the existing mental health system and what it can feel like to be in it as a service user. Chapter 3 looks at the language and terminology used in this field, its complexity, and in some cases its cruel and negative purposes and meanings, as well as how mental health service users/survivors have worked to change this.

The next chapters are concerned with developments that have challenged traditional approaches to so-called mental health. Chapter 4 focuses on the development of the survivor movement and service users' own organisations. Chapter 5 examines some of the serious inequalities that continue to operate in the mental health system and how service users/survivors and their organisations experience and seek to overcome them. In Chapter 6, we see how service users/survivors have worked together to develop their own interpretations of who they are and what has happened to them, to reclaim their identity and act together on the basis of this to bring about change. Chapter 7 focuses on one of the main areas where service users/survivors have felt change is needed. It looks at how 'mental health' issues have tended to be understood. This has largely been through a 'medical model', which many service users find damaging and unhelpful. We look at their efforts and ideas for moving to a more social understanding of 'madness and distress' and how this might help.

The final three chapters explore what policy and provision might look like if mental health services were to be based on the ideas, experience and proposals of service users/survivors and were able to cast off their narrowly medicalised inheritance. Chapter 8 sets out the kinds of principles and values that might provide the basis for such a transformed survivor-led approach to madness and distress. Chapter 9 explores the kinds of support and services that are likely to be helpful in such a survivor-led approach. Chapter 10 sets out a series of helpful routes and commitments to achieving such radical change.

The Postscript looks at some of the broader issues that face us in this 'maddening' world, and also returns to a focus on us as individuals and considers the relationship between the two.

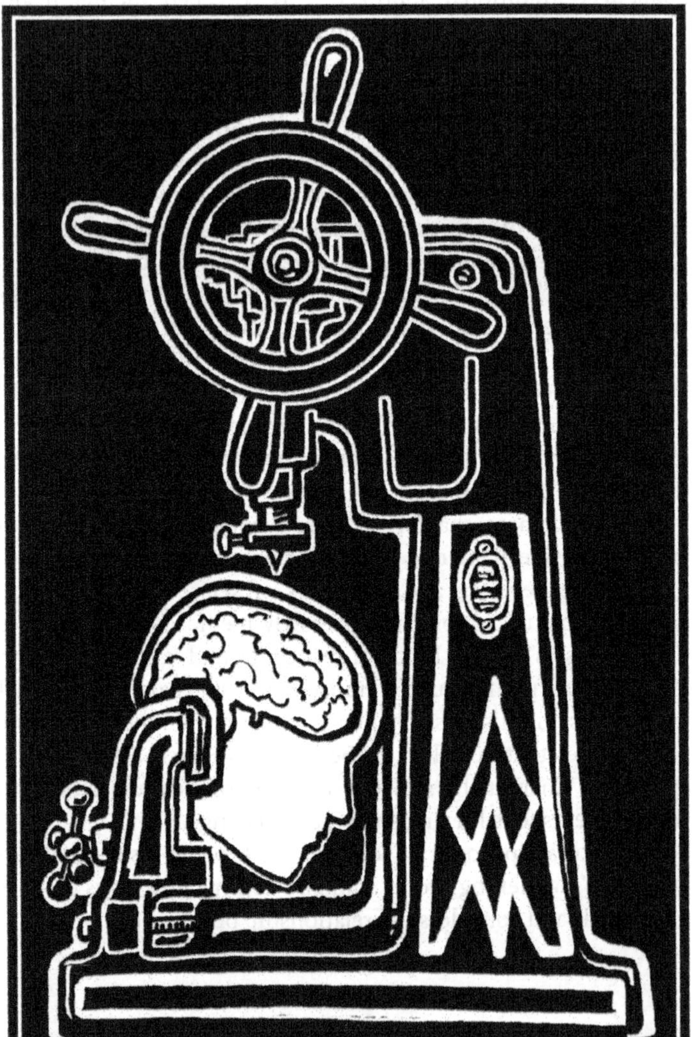

Treated like
broken machines.

Chapter 1
Setting the scene

> I know I get my strength from other service users and on my own probably couldn't do it. So, yes, I think I'm part of a movement that is saying, 'We've got something to say. We could be, we can be useful to society' and that's my feeling.
> *Discussion by group of mental health service users/survivors*

There are few things that can be said with any certainty about our lives as human beings. People's lives are all different. We have different identities, different backgrounds, different circumstances and we may want different things. But one thing does seem to be true. Nobody really wants to become a user of psychiatric or mental health services or be identified as 'mentally ill'.

How different this is to when we have a physical health problem. Of course, no one wants to be physically ill. From childhood, we learn to be wary of the taste of medicine and contact with doctors. But the health service is there for us as a safety net, somewhere to sort out our troubles and be cared for. Very often it can 'make us better'. Who thinks of psychiatric services in this way? I suspect very few, if any of us. Instead, they still seem to be the subject of a kind of folk fear – much more like the Victorian workhouse or 'lunatic asylum' than the local GP or modern hospital. We don't see them as places where we will 'get better' but as somewhere to avoid. Psychiatric services are something we hope never to have close-up dealings with, least of all for ourselves. For those of us who directly encounter such services, it can feel more like being treated as a broken machine than gaining support, understanding and care.

I remember collapsing in the street one afternoon with a panic attack. I sat, huddled against a shop window, too frightened to move until, with help, I managed to make my way to the health centre to get an emergency appointment with the GP. I didn't know what was happening to me. I was terrified. When I got there, the bureaucracy swung into action. I was told to take a seat. I sat, worried and fearful. The doctor walked through the surgery, which was empty apart from me. He had been my doctor for years and knew me. He walked straight past me without even looking in my direction. Some time passed before he called me in and I remember no helpful guidance from that consultation. That memory typified for me how the system seemed to regard people with mental health problems. It also highlighted for me the difference between bringing a physical and a mental problem to the doctors.

I have often said that I wouldn't wish my experience of mental distress on anyone except, perhaps, my worst enemy. I certainly wouldn't suggest it as a route to understanding and enlightenment. I can never get sentimental about my experience of distress or the psychiatric system. A quick think brings it all back into sharp and sometimes nasty relief. But having said that, having had to have that experience and having worked my way through it, I certainly don't wish now that it had never happened to me. I do think I have gained a better understanding of myself and other people as a result. I value the positive and sensitive professionals I have encountered. I am proud of what I have overcome and achieved. I am particularly grateful for the path it has helped set me on and for the many other people with shared and similar experience that I have got to know as a result. On balance, I believe the positive outcomes have greatly outweighed the negative ones. I suspect this may be different for many other people, especially those who have not found the support and understanding I have been fortunate enough to encounter. Of course, given the choice, I'd far rather it hadn't happened to me, far rather I had found other, gentler means of self-discovery and career guidance! But from talking to many others, I don't think my experience is unusual or the insights I have gained rare or unique.

Why am I starting by saying all this? Because I believe that, in our society, and indeed in many others, we are powerfully discouraged from talking about any experience we have of madness and distress, or letting other people know of any psychiatric experience we may have had. Many dread having to turn to such services. I know first-hand of one person who, faced with this prospect, decided to and succeeded in killing himself. He is far from an isolated instance. Many people are left on their own with secrets and difficulties that are difficult to deal with and that can overshadow their lives and their relationships.

In recent years there has been a lot of talk about 'talking about' our mental health problems: how we should feel safe being open about them and have the confidence to confide in others and challenge this 'last taboo'. Traditional mental health charities have got big money from governments and other funders to encourage such discussion. There have been 'Time to Talk' campaigns and even a 'Time to Talk Day'. Such 'anti-stigma' campaigns have become an international phenomenon. Many media stars have been drafted in to talk about the difficult times they have had in their lives and the importance of challenging traditional stereotypes. Equally, many psychiatric system survivors, including me, remain suspicious of the high-profile, non-user-led charities and governments that have sponsored such initiatives. There are some worrying contradictions in this apparently positive approach to mental wellbeing. From the introduction in the 1980s of 'care in the community' onwards, governments have been in the vanguard of those highlighting the threat of violence from mental health service users and emphasising their own commitment to prioritising the 'safety' of the public, rather than the rights of service users. In its attacks on people claiming disability benefits, the UK Department for Work and Pensions has tended to single out mental health service users for some of its most punitive and rejecting responses. These are hardly structural incentives to come out as someone diagnosed with 'schizophrenia' or 'borderline personality disorder'. As hate crime against mental health service users has continued to rise and more and more people have attempted to end their own life, or succeeded in doing so, as a result of their treatment by the Benefits Agency, the value of such anti-stigma campaigns is increasingly called into question and the need for truly effective anti-discrimination policy and legislation has more and more been highlighted.

I am a determinedly 'out' mental health service user. I don't want people not to know about my experience. This isn't about flaunting what's happened to me, making it the be-all and end-all of who I am. Rather it is about being honest and open. To be truthful, I couldn't cope without being open. I realised that some time ago, and it is why I made my personal choice. I don't want people to be hinting at things behind my back. I don't want my experience to be used or seen as some kind of vulnerability. This is how I can best cope with what happened to me. Each person will have their own way of dealing with these things. Some may want to keep them to themselves; I have friends and colleagues for whom that is the case, and I respect and understand their position. Sometimes, because of prejudices and power inequalities, it is best to be quiet about who we are. But to be truthful, I can't cope with all the secrets. I grew up with too many secrets, like my own father's suicide.

If this book and similar initiatives help one person to feel less guilty or ashamed about themselves, to feel more confident about who they are, to work through what has happened to them, to feel they don't have to have secrets unless they want to and to get to grips better with the demons they may have had, then in my mind, it has been worthwhile.

My background

One of the purposes of this book is to connect the political and the personal: the policies and practices of 'mental health' and psychiatry and the experience of being on the receiving end of them. Because of this, it seems especially important to start by saying a little about who I am and where I am coming from, so the reader can make better sense of what I say.

I used statutory mental health services over a period of 12 years. I am no longer using them, but I never assume that the need might not arise again. I don't feel that distress – mental health issues, call it what you will – is a thing of the past as far as I am concerned; rather, I am currently managing to deal with it. I know many people for whom this is true, as well as others who think of their difficulties as in the past and refer to themselves as former patients or ex-mental health service users, or perhaps don't even think of it. I can't think quite like that. I have good and bad days. Sometimes things are really hard, so I never truly feel out of the wood.

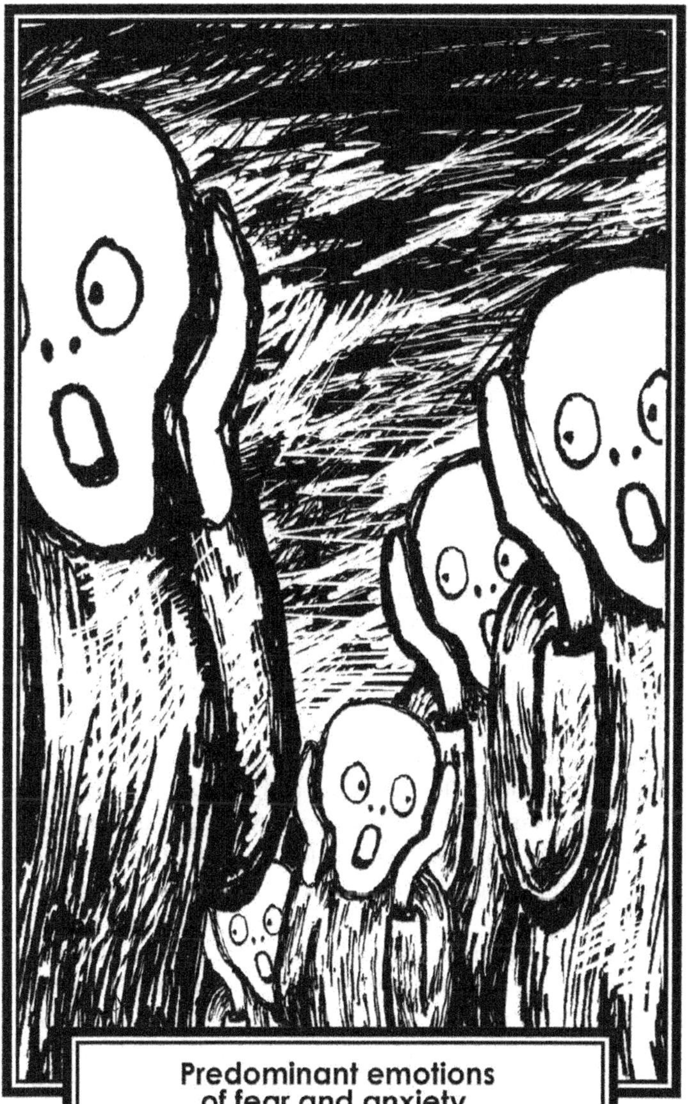

Predominant emotions
of fear and anxiety.

One of the key lessons to learn in this field is that we are all truly different. We may gain understanding from each other, but no one should assume that we are all the same; that we react the same, experience the same and that the same things work for us. Being a mental health service user, in both positive and difficult senses, really is about difference and the fact that we human beings are all different.

My experience of mental health services has involved being an inpatient and an outpatient of a psychiatric hospital, seeing psychiatrists and getting long-term support from a psychologist. It has included long term 'drug therapy' – and getting off it – as well as the involvement of many professionals, including physiotherapists, occupational therapists, nurses and social workers. It has involved group therapy and art therapy, as well as physical exercise, relaxation and breathing exercises. Some of these interventions have been helpful, others the opposite. I haven't been admitted to hospital under section or used forensic services, so there are limits to my experience. As well as using mental health services, like many others, I have lived long term – about eight years – on low-level benefits, and this for me was a difficult, worrying and painful experience. The fear of poverty lingers powerfully for me.

Poverty and distress are often associated with a constellation of other difficulties. So, like many other mental health service users, I lived for years in unpleasant, poor quality, damp and defective housing. But I was also fortunate. Unlike many, I wasn't isolated and alone. I had a family and, despite the difficulties I undoubtedly imposed on them, they stayed close and kind to me. Loneliness and isolation are terrible things, but fortunately I was spared them during my worst times.

My experience of distress has mostly been unpleasant. The predominant emotions I have experienced are fear and anxiety, although I know others who have found their experience revelatory and positive. I still have better and worse times. I still don't always understand sensations and feelings that I have. I learn more about myself and my distress all the time. But I can still find myself as confused as I have ever been by my emotions, state of mind or sense of impending disaster. I am not expecting to experience tranquillity any time soon!

Chapter 2
The psychiatric system

> Power, not illness or treatment, is what the system is all about. It is power that usually is not spoken about.
> *Judi Chamberlin (1988, p.xiv)*

The first fact that needs to be acknowledged is that the psychiatric system in a Western society like the UK is large and complex. If the issue of 'mental health' is sometimes presented in terms of something strange – a few 'weirdos' out there, far distant from the rest of 'us' – the reality is that the system exists on an industrial scale. Once it comprised enormous rural walled institutions, housing sometimes many hundreds – even thousands – of inmates in the equivalent of villages or local urban communities. They had their own laundries, shops, workshops, farms, gardens and food production, libraries, newsletters, power stations, medical centres, dispensaries, living quarters and staff residences. Frequently, they even had their own chapels and mortuaries. The modern history of mental health services has charted the run-down of such institutions.

However, the closure of the long-stay asylums does not mean that such a wide range of services and functions no longer exists. Arguably, there are now more. Nor does it mean that mental health service users/survivors aren't still segregated and separated from other people, lumped together with others seen as similar to them. There are still psychiatric hospitals and acute inpatient wards. There are medium secure units, and special hospitals (such as Rampton, Ashworth and Broadmoor). There are criminal justice diversion

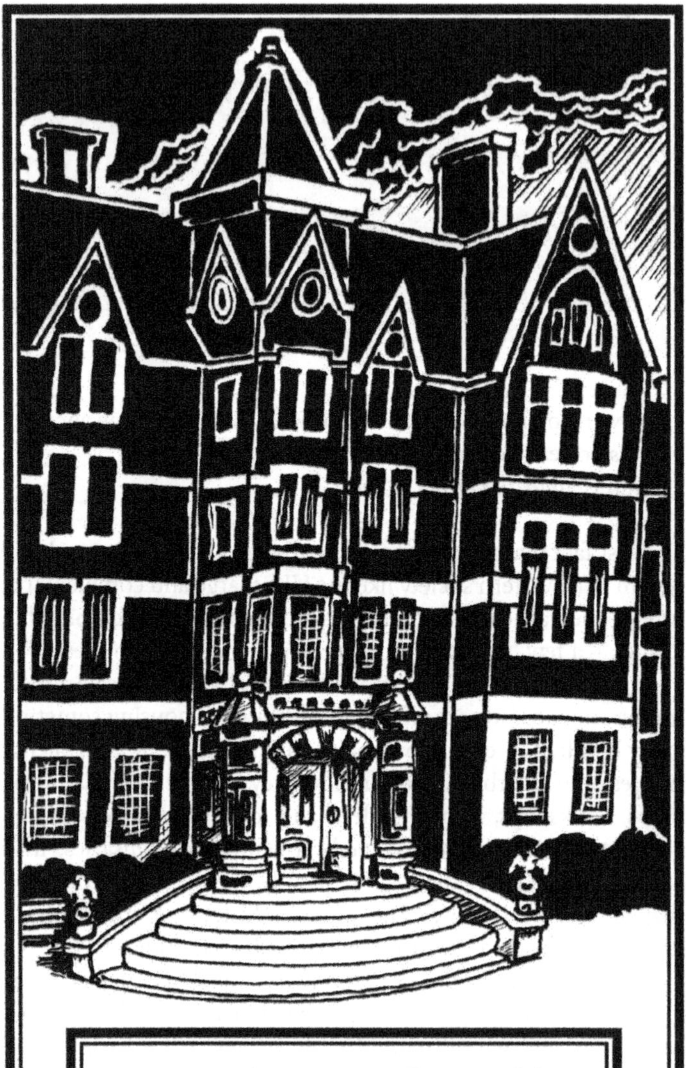

A separate segregating world.

schemes. There are day centres; day hospitals; sheltered workshops; employment schemes; crisis, home treatment, multi-disciplinary mental health and 'assertive outreach' teams; befrienders and volunteers; services for young people identified as having 'mental' or 'behavioural' problems (CAMHS), and supported housing, hostels and sheltered and so-called 'social' housing schemes. There are arts projects, gardening projects, drop-in centres, 'out-of-hours' services, therapeutic communities, 'social prescribing' schemes, helplines and social enterprises. There is almost a parallel universe of provision for people identified as needing help from mental health services.

To this must be added an even larger institutional world that is similarly a left-over from past approaches to dealing with people seen as deviant, defective or simply different. Thus, there are many mental health service users located in other sectors, such as the prison system (now often seen as serving the same institutional role as the old psychiatric hospitals), in provision for homeless people, in related services for people with alcohol and drug problems (those identified as having 'dual diagnoses'), and in residential services for older people, including those with dementia and other organic mental health problems.

Also to be included are those experiencing distress among the large numbers of asylum seekers and refugees, including children, now held in detention centres and living in hotels. They include unknown numbers traumatised by conflict, war, rape, violence and crime, who now await official decisions on their future, struggling to survive in makeshift provision for long periods, denied their human and civil rights, with their mental and physical wellbeing – often already compromised – at risk (Taylor, 2023).

It is important to highlight the scale, diversity and complexity of the UK psychiatric system, with its many different services and its wide range of professions with their different traditions, statuses and cultures. However, much stigma still surrounds the mental health system and the problems that lead people to it. It can no longer truly be seen as an isolated world, many miles distant from us, behind high walls and locked doors. Mental health services are now essentially a large, locally based system, with centres often situated alongside other health services and just a referral away from our GP. We may walk past services and facilities each day, perhaps unaware that they are part of this vast parallel world.

Yet the general feeling about the mental health system is negative, however much it has moved on from the 19th-century 'lunatic asylums'. This is not just a folk fear that arises out of ignorance and misunderstanding among people who have never had contact with it and only know it from myth and media reports. It is a commonly held view among mental health service users themselves, based on their own first-hand experience.

What it can feel like

While there is a tendency to lump mental health service users together as a homogeneous group, a more helpful generalisation is how different we may all be. What may be a problem for one may not be for another. This has certainly been one of the lessons of my experience, but it may not fit very well with a psychiatric system that has been shaped by an institutional history and what can feel like a standardising, batch approach to its clientele. This can be a poor fit with the particular situation of any individual coming its way. It can feel more like us having to adapt to the way the system works than vice versa.

This is how a long-term survivor friend of mine put it at the time of one admission when he had been very depressed. 'Dave', as I'll call him, had been labelled as a schizophrenic manic depressive with personality disorder, and much more. This was a time when he felt very down. He said:

> I felt suicidal, rubbish, nothing, useless. What I wanted was somewhere safe, somewhere where I'd be OK – sanctuary, asylum… First, they put me in the psychiatric ward of the general hospital. That was OK. Then quite quickly I was sent on to the local psychiatric hospital. It's a big, Victorian institution. [*When you speak to Dave on the patients' phone, you can hear the long corridor echoing as people walk along it.*] It's not safe. I didn't want to take things like my radio in case they were stolen. The food is rubbish.
>
> There are some good things. Other patients are a positive. The nurses are not too bad this time. Some are OK. They'll talk, but it's five minutes and then they've got to be doing something else, seeing someone else. It's the way it always is. Not enough of them.

> But when they say to me, 'You'll come through', are they saying that to me specifically? Do they mean it, or is it just what they say to patients generally? I can see them watching me to make sure I don't do anything, don't hurt myself. I have been 'specialled'. That means they follow you round, but it feels more like it's to protect them than me. There have been more [spending] cuts, even less time seeing the psychiatrists, fewer nurses, less resources and activities.
>
> Nothing really nasty has happened this time. I haven't had or seen any forced medication, verbal or physical abuse.

I met with a small group of mental health service users as part of the process of writing this book, in order to include their views. They expressed similar concerns and worries about mental health services. They focused particularly on their experience of inpatient services:

> I find that being in the psychiatric hospital is as painful as it has always been. *[General agreement]*

> ... you are given full medication and shelter, but it's all you are given... I feel that there is no psychological input. It's too much based on your medication... It feels like a prison.

> Yes, I saw a psychiatrist once every two weeks or so... But I didn't feel it was a space in which I could really voice my feelings. It was like a sitting-in-judgement situation. It didn't feel a friendly atmosphere. I found the OT [occupational therapy] department helpful. I almost consider it as something aside from life in the ward... The ward, I think it's as dreadful as it's always been... Because you're not taken care of as an individual. It is as if the fact that you are distressed – in distress – is not considered. You might find the occasional good nurse... but that's as far as it goes... Nobody's interested in you and you need so much to talk to someone and... just that opportunity was never given to me.

> Things have improved... Now you get your own room. In those days [1980s] you slept in a dormitory. You had no privacy.

> [But] the wards [there] are still very boring places... You don't get enough stimulation... A lot of people will still say that the nurses don't talk to you. They're always in the office filling in forms... They have introduced something called 'protective time' when staff are supposed to speak to you.
>
> There's a growing number of people with 'dual diagnosis' now [people using illegal drugs as well as having other diagnoses attached to them]... people with drugs, alcohol and solvent abuse... and they are much more security conscious. Video cameras for the staff to look at, at the entrances to the wards... I think it has changed for the worse... They're bringing in police with sniffer dogs at times, to see that something hasn't been brought in.

This reflects much wider comments and experience. And, whatever the picture was when this book was first written, it is generally worse now, with the cuts and lack of priority given to mental health services over the past decade and more.

A picture emerges from mental health service users/survivors of a psychiatric system that can feel frightening and strange. There can be long delays in accessing services and getting the kind of support people want. Women are still being placed in mixed wards where they feel unsafe, despite government commitment to ban the practice. The quality of acute wards continues to be highlighted in official reports as inadequate. There is a strong backlog of evidence that Black and minority ethnic service users face discrimination in mental health services and are more likely to receive controlling and coercive treatment. Service users can be put at risk from other patients who are aggressive, confused, frightened or using non-prescription drugs, without adequate staff control or supervision. Ward staff are still often poorly trained and sometimes unhelpful, abusive and aggressive. Often they retreat to their offices, rather than being available to help. There are additional problems of communication on wards where English is not the first language of many staff. High demand for beds means that service users can come under constant pressure to 'recover' and move on before they feel ready and the necessary supportive housing and other services are available.

Sadly, things are tending to get worse rather than better. There are increasing delays in getting support for people. Families can be told that CAMHS has a waiting list of 18 months to two years – by which time their child may no longer qualify for support if they are nearing the upper age limit. Some patients, including children, are being sent many miles away for treatment for want of local provision. Television documentaries are telling us about more scandals, and a growing number of patients are experiencing them directly. High-cost, privatised and for-profit services are relying on inadequately trained, poorly supported, poorly supervised and sometimes abusive staff to meet the needs of service users with complex histories and difficulties, without adequate or consistent managerial accountability (Halliday, 2022). An increasing emphasis on control and a preponderance of patients with drug and alcohol issues means that psychiatric provision has increasingly taken on the appearance of a custodial setting, with security cameras, locked doors and controlled environments – hardly a therapeutic setting conducive to holistic wellbeing.

Instead of mental health services necessarily being helpful to those attempting to deal with the difficulties and mental distress they are experiencing, they can seem like an additional obstacle they have to contend with. As 'Dave' said, when he left hospital feeling not very good at all, 'It is as if you have both your distress and the hospital to contend with.' So, the first requirement for a mental health service user can sometimes be to be able to deal with the psychiatric system itself – at a time in their life when it is probably because they are having difficulties dealing with things that they are there in the first place.

As the editors of an Open University reader on mental health matters wrote in 2009:

> Large proportions of service users and survivors who have experienced the mental health services as 'consumers' still come away dissatisfied with the way they have been treated. There are still precious few reports outside the public relations blurbs of corporate organizational literature of people having positive experiences of mental health services. (Heller & Walsh, 2009, p.272)

Sadly, if anything, the situation has grown worse since. When people talk about the NHS, when they 'clapped for the NHS' during the Covid pandemic, they were mostly thinking of the much-loved NHS for our physical health. Mental health services command little of the same affection, attention or positive response.

Yet, despite being often overlooked, the mental health or psychiatric system is not only massive, it is also complex. Its tentacles reach into many different service systems, government departments and policy frameworks. These include health, social care, housing, employment and benefits. This means that service users have to negotiate often poorly co-ordinated local authority, NHS and welfare agencies with no one to look out for them at what is likely to be a difficult time. Services may be based in the state, voluntary or private sectors. Each can be expected to have its own particular forms, routes in, officials, hierarchy, culture, ideology and ways of doing things. Service users can expect to pass and be passed between different agencies, professionals and service providers, none of which necessarily know the processes and ways of working of the others. This is anything but a seamless process, with different arrangements for assessment, different cultures and even significantly different understandings of mental health issues. Again, service users need to negotiate this, often with little help or guidance, at what might be times of extreme stress and difficulty in their lives.

It is also not only dedicated mental health services that impact on the lives of people experiencing distress and pose problems for them. The first port of call for many is their GP. As has often been observed, the majority of GP consultations relate to emotional and psychological rather than physical problems, yet often mental health service users wish they could bypass their GP because of their lack of expertise and understanding in this area. Since the Covid pandemic and continuing NHS spending cuts, the GP system – key to the functioning of the NHS – has become increasingly inaccessible and unworkable.

Mental health service users can also find that, when they have to turn to other services outside the mental health system, they are dealt with differently and get inferior treatment. Examples include the experience of people who self-harm when they access accident and emergency services, and the poor quality of care they receive from the NHS for physical health problems – 'diagnostic overshadowing', as it is called – first documented by the Disability Rights Commission (DRC) in a 'formal investigation' into the physical health inequalities experienced by mental health service users published in 2006. The same is reported of people's experience of policing. The police can be highly variable in their response and helpfulness if they are called upon to help when someone is acting in a distressed and challenging way in a public place. Some police departments have developed helpful joint initiatives with outreach health services, while others are still effectively offering only a custody and control service. Indeed, in August 2023, the Metropolitan police declared they would no longer attend 'mental health incidents' (Dodd, 2023).

It is also in such other services that issues about the stigma and stereotyping associated with being a mental health service user emerge and this can have powerful effects on people's lives and their feelings about themselves.

The dominance of 'diagnosis'

Another key point needs to be made about the psychiatric system. Everything tends to be determined by the diagnostic category in which you are placed. This shapes how you are seen, the treatment you receive and the nature of your journey through the system. It may even play a crucial role in whether that treatment is voluntary or on a compulsory basis that results in a restriction of your rights rather than you getting support for them. It is through diagnostic categorisation that the psychiatric system organises both itself and service users. Whereas treatment is the key activity through which physical health provision is understood, in the mental health sector it is diagnosis, and it is in this domain, rather than the improvement of treatment, that innovation, development and expansion have been most conspicuous.

Diagnosis is the basis for the expertise, specialist knowledge and skills that psychiatrists, the dominant psychiatric system profession, claim. Their role revolves round assessing, categorising, classifying and treating people. Not everyone knows their own diagnosis. Sometimes psychiatrists are reluctant to inform the people it most concerns – their patients – but everyone seeking help for a mental health issue is likely to have a diagnosis – quite possibly more than one – attached to them.

Many service users find their diagnosis reassuring. They feel it helps them explain and make sense of their feelings and situation. It can also validate their distress. Others reject what they see as arbitrary labels attached to them.

Diagnosis is far from an exact science. The diagnoses attached to people can change or vary, depending on the psychiatrist and with different ethnic groupings. The psychiatric system has often been accused of being 'Eurocentric' and a key expression of this seems to be the values and assumptions on which diagnosis is based. African-Caribbean young men, for example, have tended to be diagnosed disproportionately as 'psychotic' and 'schizophrenic'. The basis for diagnostic categorisation since 1952 has been the *Diagnostic and Statistical Manual of Mental Disorders* (DSM), which is published by the American Psychiatric Association and provides the diagnostic criteria for 'mental disorders'. Now in its revised fifth edition (APA, 2013), the DSM has always been contentious. One criticism is that, because it is not based on identifiable 'markers' for the various disorders it categorises, its categories reflect dominant (Western) social values – for example, for a long time it identified homosexuality as a 'disorder' and even now retains the category 'sexual orientation disturbance'.

It is also criticised (sometimes by psychiatrists) for being subjective, unreliable, inconsistent and discriminatory. Fundamentally, also, it is argued that telling people what is wrong with them is far from the same as successfully doing something about it. And psychiatry's record in that department is woeful. So the numbers of people with a psychiatric diagnosis grow exponentially, as do the numbers of categories and diagnoses in each edition of the DSM. Such poor recovery rates would be deemed completely unacceptable in the physical health services.

The development of something different

Not surprisingly, for many mental health service users, dealing with their distress and the additional difficulties they can face from receiving mental health services takes all their energy and attention. Add to this the fact that it may be happening at times of isolation, confusion and uncertainty, and few may feel in a position to analyse, let alone challenge what is happening to them. The role of 'mental patient' has long been constructed in very passive terms, with the individual questioned, categorised, 'treated' and researched, with minimal opportunities to play an active role in the process or explore what they feel or want. The effect is further to separate people from their lives and experiences, as well as the so-called 'well' population, and pathologise what can also be interpreted as natural responses to very distressing circumstances (Read & Sanders, 2022). Perhaps it is not surprising that key media images of mental health service users are of people acting strangely in some institutional, hospital or public setting, or sitting hunched over, holding their head in their hands.

Yet, despite the barriers and difficulties, the late 20th century witnessed the emergence of collective action on the part of mental health service users/survivors in the UK and internationally. It is this development that lies at the heart of this book. The lessons that the service user/survivor movement has taught us are what this book seeks to explore and share. Some of the key points that the movement has established are that there is a life during and after madness and distress; that the roots of people's so-called madness lie in their past lives and experiences; that people experiencing madness and distress are human too; that mental health service users have human and civil rights that should be respected, and that there are different and better ways of engaging with madness and distress than through traditional over-medicalised approaches.

Progress in this development has not been uniform internationally. It has been more advanced in some countries than others, and it has had different expressions in different parts of the world: for example, between the Global North and the poorer nations of the Global South.

Nonetheless, the international mental health service user/survivor movement has offered us different ways both of understanding the experience, concepts and apparatus of 'mental illness' and being a mental health service user, and of responding to madness and distress. It has also begun a process of developing new and different ideas, narratives and responses to these phenomena.

We will shortly be examining the origins of the survivor movement, but first more needs to be said about the language commonly used to define and describe 'mental health'.

Chapter 3
The language of 'mental health'

> Until there is common agreement on what is meant by 'mental illness', there can be no common language for the related concepts of patients/service users/survivors/consumers, etc... Ultimately, different people will describe themselves differently, and this is as it should be, since our movement stresses the right to self-define.
> *Jan Wallcraft & Mary Nettle (2009)*

Language in the context of 'mental health' is a field of conflict. It is almost impossible to escape this. Even my opening sentence is contentious because of the baggage that concepts like 'mental health' carry. It is hardly surprising that terminology in this field is problematic, given that it relates to what is widely seen as a stigmatising, spoiled and devalued identity – namely, using 'mental health services' and being 'mentally ill'.

There is no agreement about terminology in relation to 'mental health service users' and the 'survivor movement'. Whatever terms are used, they are likely to offend someone. My aim in this book is to try to offend as few people as possible and to be consistent with the values that generally underpin the collective action of mental health service users/survivors – of which more later. But we have to be honest and admit that language continues to be a problem in this field and it can have a damaging and divisive effect, sending out all kinds of unhelpful, if often unintended, messages. Language also has a particular importance in this field because so often it has been negative and so many of the words used to describe the experience of 'mental illness' have been judgemental and pejorative.

We have to address the issue of language without being blocked or sidetracked by it. I have encountered some professional 'experts' happy to encourage disagreements about terminology, with the effect – intentionally or otherwise – of stopping us ever getting round to working effectively together to change things! So, we may not reach a consensus about language but hopefully we can find a basis for working respectfully together, regardless of our differences.

Traditional formal language used about mental health service users/survivors has largely been rejected by service-user activists. The terms used have either followed from their role in the psychiatric system as patients or been associated with the diagnostic categories in which they have been included. Thus, the most commonly used term has been 'patient', or 'psychiatric' or 'mental' patient. Many service users/survivors reject such terms because they feel they emphasise their passivity and frame them narrowly in terms of services that they frequently dislike and reject.

People are also described in terms of diagnostic categories – such as 'schizophrenics', 'manic-depressives' or 'bipolars'. Such labels are frequently experienced as demeaning, reducing people to a set of symptoms, framing them in narrow medical terms. They are especially problematic because the diagnostic categories attached to people frequently change, overlap and do not seem to be consistently applied, and have in some cases been racialised. Such labels are especially felt to objectify and reduce the people they are attached to. Having said this, people to whom such labels have been attached sometimes use them themselves, perhaps because the labels seem to offer an explanation or justification for their situation and the difficulties they may experience. As has been said, there is no consensus here!

There is another set of terminologies that needs to be touched on too. This is the frequently derogatory, stigmatic and abusive language that is used about distress and mental health service users in popular parlance and in the media. A wide and growing range of such terms continues to be used and developed, which includes words like 'nutter', 'loony', 'nut case', 'mental case', 'mental', 'mentalist', 'psycho', 'community care case' and 'crazy'. Some can be seen as leftovers from previous ages. Others have much more recent origins. They are part of our cultural wallpaper, featuring in TV programmes for both adults and children as terms of ridicule and rejection. I have recently noticed a more enlightened popular response to disabled people generally; they tend to feature more positively in soaps and children's programmes. But being 'mental' is apparently still something for us to ridicule in adult and children's programmes on TV, as part of the background noise of our lives. It is still part of a broader environment of stigma and exclusion that mental health service users routinely encounter and that I will look at more directly later in this book.

Because the language associated with 'mental health issues' has been seen by survivors as so damaging and discriminatory, from the time that they started to develop their own groups and organisations in the 1980s, they have sought to develop their own alternatives. Two terms have been at the heart of their attempts to describe themselves. These are 'survivor' and 'service user'. The term survivor seems to have had its origins in the pioneering mental health service users' organisation Survivors Speak Out. It spoke of people as being psychiatric system survivors. The emphasis was placed on people surviving what had happened and been done to them in the psychiatric system. Others talked about mental health and psychiatric survivors, meaning people who were surviving their difficulties and distress. People also began to talk of themselves as psychiatric or mental health service users. This connected with the development of other service user organisations and movements, like those of disabled people, people with learning difficulties, those living with HIV/AIDS and older people. It was seen as offering a preferable alternative to the term 'patient'.

However, both these terms, survivor and service user, have come in for criticism. The term 'survivor' is seen as creating confusion with people who have survived domestic or sexual abuse. The term 'user' can be seen as too passive, defining people in terms of services they often do not want to receive or are even unable to access. Some people also dislike it because of its association with drug 'user'. Yet, for all their shortcomings, these continue to be the two most frequently used terms among service users/survivors. This is why I tend to use the term 'mental health service user/survivor', since it probably comes as close as we can get to reflecting the spirit of how people want to identify themselves, even if it has weaknesses of its own. This term seems to cause the least offence. I use it to mean people who currently use mental health services, or have in the past, or who would be seen as eligible to use them. There is an argument that we are all 'people' first and it is therefore unhelpful to describe ourselves distinctly as service users or survivors. But this ignores the reality for people with experience of distress and/or using mental health services – they are likely to be seen and treated as different. So, ignoring this denies their experience. The term can thus be a basis for political struggle, rather than personal objectification.

The advent of managerialism and consumerism in public policy has led to an increasing emphasis on terms like 'customer' or 'consumer'. Many survivor activists reject such terms, particularly since many mental health service users are involuntary users who are subjected to treatment under compulsory section. Mike Lawson, for example, one of the founders of the survivor movement, observed that psychiatric system survivors are 'consumers of mental health services in the same way that rats are consumers of Rentokil' (other pesticides are of course also available!). Other terms like 'service refuser' have also been developed by survivors.

Service users have also sought to move beyond prevailing medical models to describe their experiences. Thus, they have tended to talk much more about 'distress' – emotional and mental – than 'mental health' or 'mental health problems'. Some have also talked about madness, although others are uncomfortable with the term. I shall return to this when we talk about Mad Studies later in the book.

Service users have not only worked to develop their own terminology; they have also sought to reappropriate and reclaim language that has been previously used pejoratively. Thus, as we will be seeing, they have used the term 'madness' to describe differences and extremes of emotion and perception in a non-pejorative way. This can be seen as part of a broader development where mental health service users/survivors, like other oppressed groups and minorities, including Black and minoritised people, women, gay men, lesbians, bisexuals, non-binary and trans people, seek to reclaim oppressive language used against them, particularly in their communication with each other. Thus, we have seen the emergence of Mad Pride, a campaigning and activist organisation and movement committed to challenging the devalued position of mental health service users/survivors and bringing a 'mad positive' perspective to such experience and understandings.

Chapter 4
The mental health service user/survivor movement

> What underpins all this is a drive, a will to see real change for service users in terms of treatment options, of people actively participating in their care, and to make possible real social inclusion. For me it has become more than a journey of discovery or a healing process; it is also now a political engagement, an act of citizen participation.
> *Anne-Laure Donskoy (2009, p.166)*

The modern mental health service user/survivor movement is a very recent development. Its origins are usually traced to the mid-1980s. It represents a fundamental watershed in mental health issues. Yet of course many people, including many service users, don't know about this movement. This is hardly surprising, but that doesn't make it any less significant. We live in a world where the storylines of TV soaps make headline news, where people who happen to see media stars in the street think they know them because they are so used to seeing them on their phones, televisions and computer screens. Yet issues affecting the day-to-day lives of millions of people tend only to be picked up by the media if some exceptional problem, tragedy or unusual occurrence is involved that can readily be individualised.

People still frequently talk and write about 'the mentally ill' as though they were a separate group of people, very different and distant from the rest of 'us'. Discussion is still often framed in terms of what can 'we' do about 'them'. Not only does this fly in the face of the facts; it has also been well established that very high proportions of people are likely to be affected by 'mental health problems' during the course of their lives – a figure of one in four is often given. But also, most of us can expect someone close to us to have such experiences, including what are seen as the most severe and difficult problems of distress. So, although the tendency is to frame mental health issues in terms of 'other' people, and to 'other' them – that is to say, see them as inferior and alien, and later we will look at why this might be – the reality is that such experiences are much more helpfully understood as part of the human condition; something that may affect any one of us and that we can routinely expect to encounter in one way or another in our lives.

This is only the first routine inaccuracy we can expect to encounter over this issue. Another is that there is an active 'we' who are the solution and a passive 'them' who are the problem. It is unlikely that this has ever been true, but certainly over the past 30 to 40 years its truth has been challenged by the emergence of mental health service user/survivor organisations and a distinct survivor movement. The development of this movement and these organisations means that mental health service users/survivors themselves are playing an active and distinct role in doing something about mental health issues. While this role should not be exaggerated, equally it can no longer be ignored. Mental health service users, their organisations and their movement can be seen as new players in the game, bringing new ideas, knowledge, understandings, proposals and solutions to the table. So 'mental health service user/survivor' is now a term that may not only mean we have experienced being on the receiving end of mental health/psychiatric services; it is also a political identity, meaning that we actively engage with these issues from our experiences and roles in relation to the psychiatric system and beyond. I will discuss this in more detail in the next chapter.

It is this development of the survivor movement and its implications for individual mental health service users/survivors and mental health policy and practice that we want to look at in this part of the book.

The late Peter Campbell, a much-loved founding member of the UK survivors' movement, wrote of its development:

> Since 1980 the mental health system in the United Kingdom (UK) has changed dramatically. While the main types of care and treatment provided by mental health services have changed little, the location of services and mechanisms of delivery have undergone significant alteration. Simultaneously, and partly as a direct result of these transformations, those diagnosed as mentally ill, the current and former mental patients, have become more visible and vocal within society and in the corridors of power. Government seeks their views. The service provider is obliged to consult with them. (Campbell, 1996, p.218)

Peter Campbell identified much earlier examples of activism and protests by 'mad persons' from the 17th century onwards. However, he dated the modern UK survivor movement from the mid 1980s and traced its origins to earlier mental patient groups that formed early in the 1970s, and he acknowledged the support it gained from radical mental health professionals (Campbell, 2009). He also made the important point that survivors like him were more able to get engaged in this way as services became more community-based from the 1960s, rather than being segregated within long-term institutions. There has also been a developing two-way traffic of ideas and action between the UK survivor movement and its equivalents in European countries and North America. A worldwide movement now exists. There are worldwide, European, national, regional and local organisations and groups of mental health service users/survivors. As Peter Campbell noted, over an amazingly short period of time, we moved from a situation in the UK where fewer than a dozen independent user/survivor-led action groups existed to one where numbers rose probably to at least the high hundreds. Since then, sadly, cuts in funding, reactionary government public policy and years of inadequate resources have had a damaging impact on user-led organisations, but it is difficult to be precise about their numbers, since such groups and organisations do tend to come and go (Campbell, 2009, p.49).

What is also important about the survivor movement is that an increasingly wide range of people with experience of mental health services have been involved in its founding and development. They include people who have spent a long time in psychiatric hospitals, people who have spent much of their lives in and out of such hospitals, people identified as having the most serious or severe diagnoses, people who have tried to kill themselves, and people who have ongoing problems of depression, self-harm and eating distress. It has also included people who have been politically active as well as others who have never got involved before, people from many different Black and ethnic communities, men and women, older and younger people and LGBTQIA+ people.

As Peter Campbell also helpfully made clear, there is not one single position or view among people who are active in service-user/survivor organisations and the survivor movement. They may focus on different issues, have different priorities and see things in different terms (2009, p.48). But they have one thing in common that unites them and on which they tend to be agreed. All start from having personal experience of mental distress, madness and/or using mental health services. It is this direct experience, or as it is sometimes called 'experiential knowledge', that they have in common and that is their unifying force. It has been an underlying force for change in the survivors' movement as in other movements.

The mental health service user/survivor movement has not emerged in isolation. First, it needs to be understood in terms of the development of other movements of health, welfare and social care service users. These include movements of disabled people, people with learning difficulties, older people and people living with HIV/AIDS. The earliest established and best known of these is the disabled people's movement, which began to establish itself in the UK and internationally in the 1970s. While there are differences in the history, nature and objectives of each of these movements, they have some important concerns in common. All attach great importance to:

- the right of service users to speak and act for themselves
- their equal worth as human beings with other people
- the importance of their human and civil rights and needs being met.

These service-user movements also see links between themselves and other so-called new social movements (NSMs) that emerged internationally, particularly from the 1960s and 1970s, including the Black civil rights movement, the women's movement, the LGBTQIA+ movement, the older people's/grey power movement and the environmental, anti-nuclear and Occupy movements.

What distinguishes many of these movements is that they have grown out of the sense of oppression and discrimination felt by the groups who established them. They represent determined efforts to speak and act on their own behalf – to 'self-organise' – and develop aims, ideas, ways of working and cultures of their own to achieve their own self-defined goals (Jordan & Lent, 1999; Lent, 2002). These are movements that are based on identity and lived experience, and people's efforts to define their own. Identity and lived experience are key issues in relation to mental health service users/survivors and we will return to this shortly.

These movements also represent a new politics that is not confined narrowly to people's material situation or class and economic relations – important though these are. They connect closely with ways in which people are excluded, marginalised, oppressed and discriminated against. They are also linked with concerns about broader issues, like the environment, peace and nuclear weapons. All have been concerned with developing new approaches to involvement, diversity and the extension of democracy beyond formal and bureaucratic structures and approaches. Each has developed its own culture or cultures.

The same has been true for service user movements. They have been more than just organisationally based. To enable the involvement of people who traditionally had often been excluded from political and collective involvement, all have highlighted the development of new more inclusive and accessible ways of organising, new ways of doing things, new kinds of culture and arts, the development of new knowledges, new ideas and different forms of communication and expression.

Empowerment

Some people, as has been seen, view service-user movements like the survivor movement as 'new social movements'; others see them as liberatory movements, and there has been much academic discussion about this. Whichever interpretation is placed upon

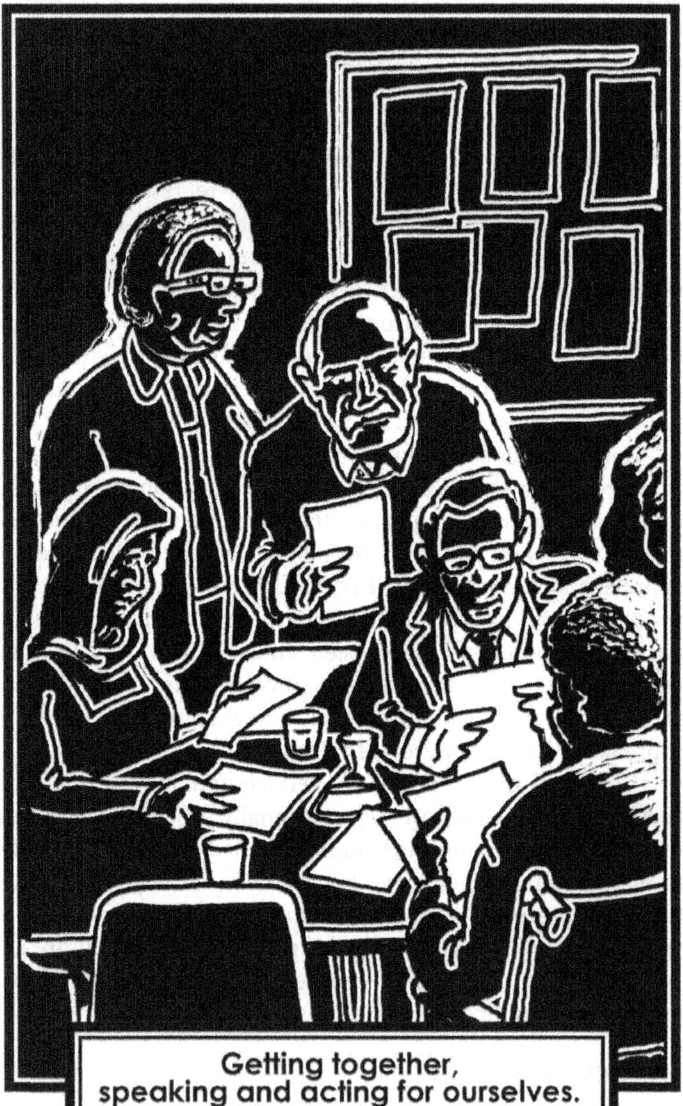

Getting together,
speaking and acting for ourselves.

them, however, there seem to be two important and interrelated things that such movements do. These are:

1. Provide opportunities for people to get a better understanding of themselves and gain personal and practical skills
2. Work together to achieve broader political and social change.

Key commentators of these movements, like Mike Oliver in the mental health world and Vic Finkelstein of the disabled people's movement, have stressed that working together, or taking 'collective action', is the best route to achieving both of these. In our society, there is a lot of emphasis on 'self-help', with books, videos, apps, podcasts and programmes about how people can turn their lives around and become more assertive or 'successful' by doing things individually, on their own (Oliver, 1996). A crucial principle of such movements, including the mental health survivor movement, is that we are much more likely to achieve such change – in ourselves and beyond – by getting together with other people. Over the past 70 years or so, a new concept has developed that embodies this view. It is called empowerment. Although the term is often used in vague and unclear ways and has lost some of its power and value as a result, it is still very helpful.

First popularised by the Black civil rights movement of the 1950s and 1960s in the USA, what it highlights is that making social and political change is inseparable from making personal change. One is unlikely to happen without the other. So, empowerment as a radical idea is concerned with:

- making change within ourselves as a basis for...
- ... working together from this position to make broader societal change (Shera & Wells, 1999).

Both are essential, and the belief is that, if political change is truly to be inclusive and democratic, then we will all need to be involved in the process, and a process of personal growth and development will also need to take place within each of us to make this possible. Otherwise, we are likely to end up as just a stage army, rather than a true mass movement.

Service user/survivor organisations

We have seen the development of many different kinds of service user/survivor organisations, big and small, doing different things. Some focus particularly on offering mutual aid and support, others are more concerned with campaigning and activism, while others are concerned with both. Both aims are valued in service-user organisations, as are the interrelations between them. Some organisations are democratically constituted, with written constitutions; others are more informal. Some are closely bound up with services and work to help people who are currently in such services, and may owe their origins to enthusiastic professionals who helped initiate them. Others provide services themselves. Some are closely linked with traditional charitable organisations; others are more determinedly independent. Some longstanding voluntary organisations, like Mind and Together for Mental Wellbeing, have developed internal user groups or sections.

There are networks, user groups and organisations for people with particular experiences and diagnoses – for example, people who hear voices, who self-harm or have been given a diagnosis of 'bipolar disorder' or 'schizophrenia'. Others are organised around issues of difference: for example, for and of Black and minority ethnic mental health service users, women or lesbians. We have seen the development of user groups operating in hospitals and services, as well as in communities and linked with day and other services.

The many local organisations and groups of mental health service users/survivors can be seen as the movement's lifeblood. They can take many forms, providing a base both for activism and mutual support. As Mary Nettle, a longstanding survivor activist and researcher, has said:

> The user/survivor movement cannot exist without a place for people to meet and swap experiences; this often starts with being an inpatient in hospital and carries on outside hospital settings, often run by well-meaning voluntary organisations which often have the same attitudes as are found in hospital. However they can be a catalyst for people who want more than just a cup of tea and a chat and it can then become a safe

> place to discuss what could be better about the mental health system locally. In order to do this, information is shared and a group may be formed. People may want to know more and find out or are told about national user/survivor groups. Some are safe, like Mindlink within Mind, others more challenging, such as the late-lamented Survivors Speak Out. People can then begin to spread their wings but in my view need to have support to be just a user/survivor at grassroots level. (Personal communication)

While a number of national organisations of mental health service users/survivors have been established – perhaps most significantly, Survivors Speak Out, the United Kingdom Advocacy Network (UKAN), and more recently, the National Survivor User Network (NSUN) – these have tended to face particular problems of funding, security and in some cases credibility, as Peter Campbell has also suggested (2009, p.48). While of course in terms of overall numbers of people with experience of distress or using mental health services, the numbers involved in service user organisations can be seen as quite small (and although there are no accurate figures, they have certainly numbered in the thousands), this is an unprecedented development, at both personal and political levels. These are people who in the past would neither have had the opportunity, nor in all likelihood ever have expected, to be actively involved alongside other people with similar experience. By doing so, they challenge other people's and their own expectations of themselves. This says a lot about what mental health service users/survivors are capable of – given the chance. In the next section we will look more closely at the status and identity of mental health service users/survivors in order to highlight even further the great leap forward this development of collective action and the survivor movement represents.

Earlier, we heard from Mary Nettle, a survivor activist and researcher. She was also for some time the Chair of the European Network of (ex-)Users and Survivors of Psychiatry (ENUSP). As she makes clear, while many barriers remain, survivors and their movement are now operating on an international scale as well as being fuelled by the strength of their grassroots organisations:

> It is possible to move from grassroots to national to European and international within the user/survivor movement more easily than you would think. All it needs is the will to want to look further than your own situation and the support to see that it is possible. Resources are always an issue as user survivors are amongst the poorest members of society, and a broadband Internet connection in your own home now makes communication and knowledge exchange so much easier. The reality of living with a psychiatric label is what binds us together despite cultural and legal differences. The work on the UN Convention of Rights of People with Disabilities has led to a treaty which will make a difference to our lives as user/survivors when we are informed by our peers in the international movement WNUSP (World Network of (ex-)Users and Survivors of Psychiatry) and backed up at the European level by ENUSP (European Network of (ex-)Users and Survivors of Psychiatry). Both organisations struggle for resources and rely on voluntary effort and some membership fees to exist. Both manage to get people together for occasional general assemblies to ensure that they are more than just a virtual body joined by the Internet. (Personal communication)

It would be wrong, though, to suggest that the picture overall has been one of uninterrupted progress. Instead, more recently in particular, and certainly in the UK, the opposite has been true. This has been related to the strengthening hold of new-right, neoliberal ideology in mainstream UK government politics. Before lockdown, two national user-led organisations, Shaping Our Lives and the National Survivor User Network (NSUN), came together to examine the evidence. They found that a large and growing number of such user-led organisations were having to close or their situation was becoming more tenuous and uncertain because of funding cuts and the pattern of funding distribution. They also identified that, while user-led organisations have been shown to be particularly valued by service users/survivors, a disproportionate amount of state and non-statutory funding was still being directed to the large, traditional, non-user-led charities like Mind, Rethink and others. The two user-led organisations brought together funders and other user-led groups to discuss the crisis at a national meeting and highlight the serious nature of the problem (Beresford, 2019). However, at the time of writing, little has been done more generally to improve the underlying situation. The high visibility of traditional charities, the legitimacy granted to them, their reluctance to 'rock the boat' and their greater power means that they are able to overshadow local user-led organisations. Meanwhile, their general preparedness to continue to be uncritical of government policy in order to secure service contracts and maintain their privileged position has protected them significantly from austerity and small-state policies that run strongly counter to the rights and interests of mental health service users and other disadvantaged groups.

The negative impact of Covid-19

Despite the progress that has been made by the survivor movement, user involvement in the UK can often feel like taking two steps forward and then one step back. Nothing illustrates this so powerfully as the Covid-19 pandemic and the policy response of the UK government. If anything has highlighted the importance of a participatory approach to policy generally and to mental health issues specifically, it is this pandemic. Different countries approached this public health threat in different ways, some far more successfully than others. Sadly, the UK was among those, like the US and Brazil, with some of the least successful responses. At the height of the pandemic, the UK was one of the most badly affected countries in Europe – among comparable higher-income countries, only Spain and Italy reported greater numbers of deaths. Across the world, countries such as New Zealand and South Korea, where far more effective, less ideologically-led policies operated, reported much lower rates.

UK Covid policy can be seen as a case study of the failings of non-participatory, ideologically-driven approaches to policy development. It also has particular relevance to mental health service users/survivors and associated policymaking. The first thing to make clear is that this was a pandemic that affected the worst-off, the least powerful and the most vulnerable. Compromised health and immunity, living with long-term health conditions, poverty, poor housing and poor quality, low-paid employment were all strongly associated with susceptibility to the virus. And groups associated with such characteristics, like Black and minoritised people, older and disabled people and mental health service users, were all also at particular risk (Williams et al., 2021).

But there was also another big issue here. Groups like mental health service users were in a particularly helpful position to offer insights and understandings from their own day-to-day experience to help policymakers ensure that the actions they took to contain the pandemic did not make things worse in other ways. Routine experience of isolation, loneliness and being restricted to within their own four walls meant that many mental health service users had valuable intelligence to offer about managing social distancing, lockdowns, working at home, virtual living and the rest. Their experiential knowledge could have saved much psychological damage and enabled better decisions to be made about trade-offs in relation to risks of infection and mental health. Yet, as has been officially acknowledged, there was an effective halt to much vaunted public/patient involvement (PPI) programmes during the pandemic, as if a serious national emergency could not be bothered with such 'superficial add-ons'. This gives us some idea of official thinking on the subject and is likely to have added significantly to both the human and policy costs of this public health and research emergency (NHS Health Research Authority, 2021).

Chapter 5
Mental health services and inequality

> Black service users/survivors think that there is an emerging Black movement but it is very fragmented at the moment. There is a need for groups to come together to support and sustain one another and some evidence shows this is beginning to happen. But the people we spoke to find they are often not supported by larger organisations that could help them with funding and other resources, and Black service users/survivors who are working hard to raise awareness often end up feeling unheard, unvalued and exhausted.
> *Jan Wallcraft, John Read & Angela Sweeney (2003, p.39)*

Madness, mental distress and using mental health services tend not to be valued in Western societies such as the UK. Instead, we can expect the opposite kind of response. As with other aspects of life, there have been some recent attempts to associate mental health problems more positively by inviting celebrities to talk publicly about their own struggles. But as one mental health service user has written:

> Bipolar disorder is often 'glamorised' these days by its association with creative types such as Stephen Fry, but my own experience of the illness is far from that. (Howley, 2009)

Although we hear of other societies where madness and distress are valued and celebrated, it is difficult to find examples of this in modern Western societies. Of course, sometimes issues associated with distress and madness, like hearing voices, self-harm or suicide, are highly regarded, but in those cases they tend to be linked with other situations, qualities or values that mean they are accorded a status that would not ordinarily be extended to mental health service users/survivors. Such phenomena, like seeing visions and hearing voices, are, for example, associated with many religions and expressions of spirituality, from Christian saints to shamanism.

Links between 'mental health problems' and inequality are well established (Gomm, 2009). Thus, people generally expect to be seen in a negative light if they are associated with 'mental health problems'. What's more, groups already experiencing discrimination and oppression also tend to be regarded more negatively and to be treated worse. In this way, the mental health system and madness and distress have been strongly linked with inequality and the devaluing of difference. Indeed, the psychiatric system can be seen as one that has worked to reinforce and enforce conformity and to undermine and reject diversity. Thus, people from marginalised groups that face material and social disadvantage and discrimination in society may be more likely to come to the attention of the psychiatric system and then to face more difficult experiences if they do.

This seems to happen in relation to all forms of difference, including diversity in gender, sexuality, ethnicity, belief, class, age, disability, culture and so on (Sayce, 2000; Gomm, 2009). A sad reality of the psychiatric system seems to be that it reflects and reinforces broader discriminations, rather than challenges them. Age is one that is less often mentioned: young people seem particularly poorly served by mental health services, while older people appear to be at particular risk of receiving inferior, poor quality services and support, if they receive any. Yet older people are a group with high rates of organic mental illness, in the form of dementia. We should also remember that suicide is one of the leading causes of death among young and older people.

We will look at three areas of discrimination in particular, but this should not be taken to mean that the problems identified are unique or exceptional to these cases.

Sexuality

Linda McFarlane (1998), in a qualitative study of lesbians, gay men and bisexuals in mental health services, concluded that, while negative responses to their sexuality had an impact on the mental health of most participants, they did not have equal access to mental health services, the quality of the response to them was patchy, lack of safety was an urgent issue, discriminatory attitudes were pervasive and mainstream services needed 'vast improvement'. She evidenced high levels of homophobia within the mental health services, showing how this further exacerbated the distress experienced by users.

In 2018, in a report on physical and mental health in the LGBTQIA+ community in Britain, the campaign group Stonewall painted an even more disturbing picture of high levels of discrimination, exclusion and poor treatment in the mental health system (Stonewall, 2018).

Patsy Staddon (2005) identifies as a mental health service user/survivor and has long-term experience of homelessness and using alcohol. She has written about the experience of lesbians within the mental health system and the research exploring the problems facing them, which she summarises thus:

> Most lesbians I have spoken to attempt to conceal their sexual identity in treatment, so it is not well documented although Busfield [2006] has pointed out that 'severe mental health problems may themselves result from the infringement of human rights'. Depression and anxiety are believed to be common among lesbians and caused by homophobia... Bent and McGilvy [2006] produced evidence that such depression is likely to result from feeling different, fearing the consequences of sexual orientation becoming known, either while a child or as an adult in the workplace, and feeling unable to share personal details such as loss of a partner. Lesbians without good support are particularly likely to kill themselves, due to depression and isolation. These issues were also evidenced in my own research.
>
> Being a member of a minority is stressful and lesbians more than heterosexual women tend to feel the ill effects of a value system based on a heteronormativity. This is

> especially true for those who have felt unable to live open lives. Homophobia creates depression, a major factor among women who misuse alcohol… Lesbians can become unhappy and depressed because of their families' incomprehension of their lesbianism, their inability to share in the lives of heterosexual workmates and their being ignored by the health providers and educators. If the lesbian scene is not for them, they may experience loneliness. (Staddon, 2005)

Patsy Staddon's discussion highlights the particular difficulties facing lesbian women, especially in relation to the intersections between mental distress, their sexuality and 'treatment' responses. The Stonewall research updates and adds to this data for the LGBTQIA+ community more generally, highlighting higher rates of depression, anxiety and suicide in a situation of deteriorating mental health services and support (Stonewall, 2018).

Mary O'Hagan, a New Zealand activist survivor, offers further insight that relates again to the state of the international survivor movement. Active in both lesbian and survivor campaigning, she concludes:

> I sometimes think if I'd joined the gay rights movement as a young woman I might have felt happier than I do today because so much has changed for lesbian and gay people in countries like ours. I'm not very happy about the progress we have made in the 'mad' movement and I've experienced a lot of sadness and anger about it. If I talked to a young person today who wants to change the mental health system, I'd probably warn them that they might end up at my stage of life wondering what difference they made. (O'Hagan, 2022, pp.30–31)

Trans issues

Since the first edition of this text was published, the rights of transgender people, the gender binary and the whole issue of being a trans person have become increasingly contentious and headline news. The narrow politicisation of these issues by some of their ideological opponents has meant that this has tended to generate as much heat as light and sometimes more hostility and division than understanding and equal acceptance. One consequence has been to create an increasingly destructive atmosphere for those seen as challenging the status quo, as well as creating more difficult and demanding processes for them to have to negotiate. All this needs to be put in the context of the mental health difficulties that trans people are more likely to face, the increasing demand for support and ever-decreasing public resources, and the tendency within the mental health system, as well as more widely in society, to confuse identity issues around transitioning and gender with 'mental disorder', and their consequent, frequently unhelpful framing in psychiatric terms (Hill, 2016; Brooks, 2022).

Ethnicity and race

The treatment of Black people and members of minority ethnic groups in the psychiatric system mirrors and makes worse the wider discriminations that they face (Mental Health Foundation, 2021). African-Caribbean and African people, for example, are over-represented in psychiatric institutions. They are most likely (along with Irish people) to be kept on locked wards and to be given higher doses of potentially hazardous medication than are other groups and are more likely than other ethnic groups to be diagnosed with schizophrenia. African-Caribbean people, particularly young men, are more likely to come into the mental health services via the criminal justice system than to be referred through the more usual routes such as GPs or social services. They are more liked to be 'treated' with medication, rather than offered talking therapies, and to be subject to coercive measures, and are also over-represented in special hospitals, medium secure units and prisons.

While it is important not to over-simplify, particularly across different ethnic groups, the evidence continues to show that mental health services are not adequately meeting the needs of Black and minority ethnic (BME) communities because they are not sufficiently sensitive or responsive to the diversity of culture, needs and experience, and that these groups have little confidence in them (Bansal et al., 2022). While the government has not accepted this, concerns have been expressed at the highest levels that mental health services are 'institutionally racist'.

Psychiatric structures of inequality

The racism that has extended deeply into the Western approach to mental wellbeing and the psychiatric system has also recently been more closely associated with a constellation of associated racist ideas, practices and traditions. These extend from colonisation and the subordination of indigenous peoples to assumptions of white privilege and institutionalised racism. All of these are now being challenged for their historically inherited racist assumptions and inequalities, as well as their perpetuation of inequalities of power, wealth and opportunity, extending into the formulation of knowledge, education and learning, professional practice, ideology, policy and politics (King, 2022).

All of these problems may be found wherever psychiatry has been imposed on and exported to subject societies and groups. Countries like New Zealand, Australia and Canada are still grappling with the exploitative and disempowering consequences of colonisation for their indigenous peoples. So too are others, like India and African nation states, where Western psychiatric understandings and institutional systems have been imposed, overlaying and corrupting their peoples' indigenous understandings of madness and distress.

In the UK, the Black musician and footballer David 'Rocky' Bennett died while being forcibly restrained in psychiatric hospital in 1998. An independent inquiry team was set up to investigate, which reported in 2004. The chair of the inquiry identified Bennett's death as being due to institutional racism (Carvel, 2004). Yet efforts to deny this have continued ever since, and were sparked off again in 2023 by the finding of the Casey Review that the Metropolitan Police were similarly institutionally racist.

Patricia Chambers, a service user/survivor and researcher and activist, worked as a project manager in mental health for a BME health organisation. She said:

> Being Black and in the psychiatric system is bad for your mental health. You're not taken as seriously having a problem until the situation has escalated to the stage where you've hurt yourself or someone else. Quite often the only way to survive the mental health system is to 'do your own thing' within it

> and hope you don't get caught. We are coming into the system at three times the rate of other racial groups. We are more likely to be restrained when in the system than any other racial group and more likely to be given medication rather than talking therapy and we are making up the majority of patients on the locked and secure wards and the average stay on the secure wards is ten years and the cherry on the top of the cake is that you can also lose your life in the mental health system. Something that, if you're Black, you're very much aware of. Where are the white David 'Rocky' Bennetts or Orville Blackwoods? The picture is very bleak and yet we are expected to entrust our precious brains, intellect and spirit to a system that is failing us. And we know it. (Personal communication)

Sadly, Patricia ended her own life after making a massive contribution to supporting Black survivors and to the survivor movement. Today, refugees and asylum seekers form an emerging particularly vulnerable group because of the trauma and loss they have frequently experienced. We have seen their situation worsen as their access to benefits and services has been further restricted and media campaigns and aggressive political policies have increased the stigma and hostility that they are subjected to. Black people and minority ethnic groups are still under-represented in service user/survivor groups and organisations, despite growing efforts to be more inclusive. While they have established their own local and national self-help and self-advocacy organisations, these often face particular difficulties maintaining their independence and securing and keeping funding, and as a result have often struggled to survive (Beresford, 2000; Browne, 2009).

Jenny Morris, writing from a disabled woman's perspective, has cast helpful light on how the oppressive nature of mental health services can be expected to interact with other inequalities and discriminations:

> As far as the question of whether it is 'gender or disability', or indeed 'race or sexuality' which are the more important determinants of experience, I don't find this way of looking at our lives very helpful either. I think this is partly because our

> experiences are not fragmented into analytical categories. When Ayesha Vernon interviewed other Black and ethnic minority women, she found that 'Disabled Black and ethnic minority women experience a multiplicity of barriers resulting from the combination of disability or gender which determine their experiences, as one of them put it, 'it happens singularly, plurally and multiply, and it's the totality that counts at the end of the day. You are completely thought of as inferior because you are all three things.' (Morris, 1996, p.3)

This is likely to apply equally to mental health service users/survivors where the discriminatory effects of such provision operate in complex interaction with other broader inequalities and discriminations in society, imposing negative identities on people and reinforcing stigma and destructive stereotypes. This connects with the important issue of intersectionality (of which more later): that is, the way our multiple identities interact with each other in complex ways – for example, a woman may be a Black mental health service user who is also a lesbian, a mother, and older.

This brings us to our next key concern and the next chapter, which addresses how the survivor movement has helped people challenge the negative identities imposed on them as users of mental health services.

Chapter 6
Issues of identity

> My ‘recovery’ from persistent suicidal feelings came about through spiritual self-enquiry after all the psycho-medications and talking therapies had failed and sometimes made things worse. Following this spirit of enquiry, it now seems fairly natural (though blessed with much good luck) that, before long, I found myself doing a doctorate looking into the first-person perspective on suicidality. Doing a doctorate has been its own extraordinary journey and adventure.
> *David Webb, (2009, p.170)*

We have seen how using mental health services can add to your difficulties and be widely stigmatising. In societies like ours, being a mental health service user has long been what sociologists call having a ‘spoiled identity’. Few would want to identify as having used mental health services. Most people want to keep it to themselves. They expect others to shy away if they find out. Such a status is likely to have a seriously damaging effect on anyone’s self-image, hopes and life chances.

However, this has begun to change fundamentally. I am not talking here about the efforts that are more broadly being made to challenge negative public views of mental health service users. I am referring specifically to the efforts of service users themselves, particularly over the last 40 or so years, to rethink who they are – to ‘reclaim’ their identity, or identities. Clearly this is a slow business, but this is a new and important development in the history of our mental wellbeing.

Of course, we can guess that, over the years, many people experiencing madness, distress and the psychiatric system have tried to make sense of what is happening to them and have developed their own understandings and interpretations of their feelings and emotions. There is a large and influential literature of such writings by and about people with such experience, ranging from Sylvia Plath's *The Bell Jar*, to Ken Kesey's *One Flew Over the Cuckoo's Nest*. The development of the survivors' movement and the opportunities it has provided for people to come together in groups and organisations have, however, been central in enabling mental health service users/survivors to reflect on and reassess their identity and challenge dominant versions and accounts of it.

Being a mental health service user

While it may in popular imagination conjure up some very rigid stereotypes, the identity of 'mental health service user' actually embraces a very wide range of people, circumstances and experiences. Talk to people involved in a service-user organisation or group and you can expect to meet a wide range of mental health service users. They are likely to include people who have spent years in psychiatric hospital, who have had numerous 'breakdowns', who have been subject to compulsory sections and who have spent much of their life living on medication and poverty-level benefits. Expect them to include people in employment as well as people who have found the labour market too difficult to work in; people who are or have been homeless or in the prison system, and people who have 'severe and enduring mental illness' and have had every kind of psychiatric diagnostic label attached to them. There will be people who fit negative media stereotypes of 'loner' because of their isolation and breakdown of relationships, as well as people living with partners and families, bringing up children and supporting others. There will also be service users who have made every effort to keep out of the system as best they can for years, but for whom it still looms large in their life because of their fears of coming into contact with it again.

Who are we?

Each of us at some point or points in our life is likely to think, 'Who am I?' It is one of the big questions human beings ask. Why am I here? What is the meaning of life? Where do we all come from and where are we heading? We may think about our identity in relation to our family and others, in relation to the past, or with hopes and plans for the future. People sometimes talk about 'reinventing' themselves. Each of us has fixed elements making up our identity: for example, the period in which we live, the gender officially assigned to us, ethnicity, country of origin and so on. But as well as these external realities, there are also all the subjective issues of how we see ourselves and, indeed, how others see us. We hear of famous and beautiful people who have always been unhappy with their looks. We come across talented and important people who feel imposters and failures.

When we experience distress, a breakdown or a 'mental health problem', it can be catastrophic, shattering and unprecedented. It can be difficult to think it through carefully, to try to take stock and reflect. That's certainly how it was for me. We may be in turmoil. We may have little to go on. It's quite likely that if anybody else we know has had similar things happen to them, they won't have talked about them. If we turn for help to popular discussions of madness or distress, or what the 'experts' tell us, our anxieties may be increased rather than reduced. For most of us, having a 'mental health problem' is something cataclysmic to our sense of self and we may have little equipment to deal with it.

Given this, it is not surprising that many mental health service users are glad to have a diagnostic label attached to them, which at least suggests that their experience is not unique and unprecedented, that someone has got the measure of it, even if such labelling can be frightening and stigmatising. The likelihood is that we will 'internalise' prevailing views of 'people like us'. We will see ourselves as others see us: 'ill', 'sick', 'non-functioning', devalued and different – and perhaps a little alarming. Superimposing this mindset on all the issues that may go with our experience of distress is only likely to make it more difficult for us to deal with and escape assumptions and preconceptions about us and our possible future.

Identity – traditional approaches

For a long time, people who use psychiatric or mental health services have been talked about as a distinct and separate group. This has reflected their segregation and separation in society. While terms have changed, this has been a constant. So, we have had 'lunatics', 'the insane', 'the mentally disordered', 'the mentally ill' and 'people with mental health problems'. The last two terms are still frequently used. Labels have become more euphemistic, but they denote the same devalued category. Such terms have been linked with the language, institutions and systems by which people have been understood and defined. Talk of people as 'neurotic' and 'psychotic' has entered vernacular language. People have also commonly been described by the diagnostic labels that are attached to them: for example, as 'schizophrenic', 'bipolar', 'manic depressive' and so on. As I have said, it is difficult to avoid internalising these identities and seeing yourself in these terms too. After all, this is the prevailing way in which people may be defined in society. It can be difficult to keep at bay. We can be a parent, a partner, husband, wife, worker and much more. But suddenly it can all be reduced to being 'a mental health service user'. This can take over from other things and become people's defining identity, and in a way that doesn't happen for someone who needs treatment for a physical health problem. And of course, as we have already seen, this is a negative identity to be defined by. Given that we are unlikely to be in a 'strong' state if and when this happens to us, it is not surprising if our resistance to such interpretation is weakened.

However, the emergence of the survivor movement and survivor organisations has at last given people the chance to think again about their situation and their identity – in association with others who have gone through similar experiences.

Defining our own identities

Getting together in groups provides a chance for service users to have safe discussions with others who have been through similar situations without feeling judged, without having to worry what others will think of them, without the assumption that they must be 'mad' or 'weird' or 'strange'. It can make it possible for them, perhaps for the first time, to talk freely and openly about what they have been through. They don't have to deal with assumptions that it's 'all their own fault', or that 'something's wrong with them'. People can at last be in a position and feel able to analyse the system that has constantly analysed them. Its analysis of them, whatever its intention, has too often seemed condemnatory. It has felt judgemental, constantly reinforcing views of them as defective, inferior or even deviant.

Ironically, although the psychiatric system has been strong on such analysis, this has not often served as the starting point for effective intervention and improvement. It might offer a powerful system of analysis – one that can frequently feel crushing to those included within it – but the evidence is that this has not necessarily provided the basis for valued, reliable and effective responses, or 'treatments'. Modern physical medicine, by contrast, has been characterised by its increasing ability at least to ameliorate and sometimes to cure conditions that originally were seen as irrevocable and fatal, from cancer and tuberculosis to HIV and childhood leukaemia. In the last few years, physical medicine has pioneered keyhole surgery, surgery by robot and surgery on foetuses, artificial hearts, transplants and much more. There isn't the same pattern of innovation in mental health policy and provision.

The emergence of the survivors' movement has made it possible for service users to gain different understandings of themselves and place different interpretations on their circumstances and experience. Even where this does not happen, it has made it possible to gain hope and raised expectations through seeing what other service users in similar circumstances have managed to do. It has truly given people the chance to rethink in positive terms who they are and what they might be.

This doesn't mean that all mental health service users/survivors will see themselves as the same or in the same way. Not everyone will necessarily feel pride in being mad or want to attach such a word to themselves. Some of us may still feel weighed down and restricted by our experience of madness or distress. Imposing orthodoxy on how we see ourselves is unlikely to be any more helpful than having other people do the same thing to us. What does become more possible is for us not to have to blame ourselves for our situation or see it solely in terms of something wrong with us or that we have done wrong. It makes it possible to recognise the broader relations of such experience and that it neither invalidates us as people in our own right nor means that achievements, successes and indeed happiness will inevitably be beyond any of us and pass us by.

Identity politics

This reconception of who we are – our identity and experience – and the recognition that we are part of something bigger and collective, have been made possible by the emergence of the survivor movement and also form a key foundation on which the movement is built. This is what is sometimes described as identity politics, where who we are and our associated experience are key to our political viewpoint, both shaping and unifying it. This tends to be defined in terms of political arguments and approaches that are based on self-identified social minority and social interest groups, usually associated with being marginalised or oppressed.

As we have said, such 'new social movements' are significantly different to traditional social movements, which are generally based on our relationship with work and the economy, our class position and economic interests. They make for a more nuanced and complex analysis that does not ride roughshod over other forms of discrimination and inequality that have tended to operate unchallenged in societies – beyond and in addition to class and economic differences.

What mental health service users/survivors have in common is their experience – both of distress and responses to it – and the resulting experiential knowledge that is born of this. That is the basis of their movement. That shapes its focus and underpins its politics. It is the same with other liberatory groupings, such as the Black civil rights movement, the feminist movement and the LGBTQIA+ movement. All these groups of people have come together and act politically together on the basis of who they are and the resulting oppression and discrimination they have faced. What distinguishes such movements is that their members start by redefining themselves on their own terms, rather than accepting other people's historically biased and negative understandings of them. Psychiatric system survivor is both a personal and a political identity. Survivors are unified by their experience of distress and of a psychiatric system and broader society, both of which they experience as oppressive. Their politics are closely based on the personal as well as the political, unifying the two.

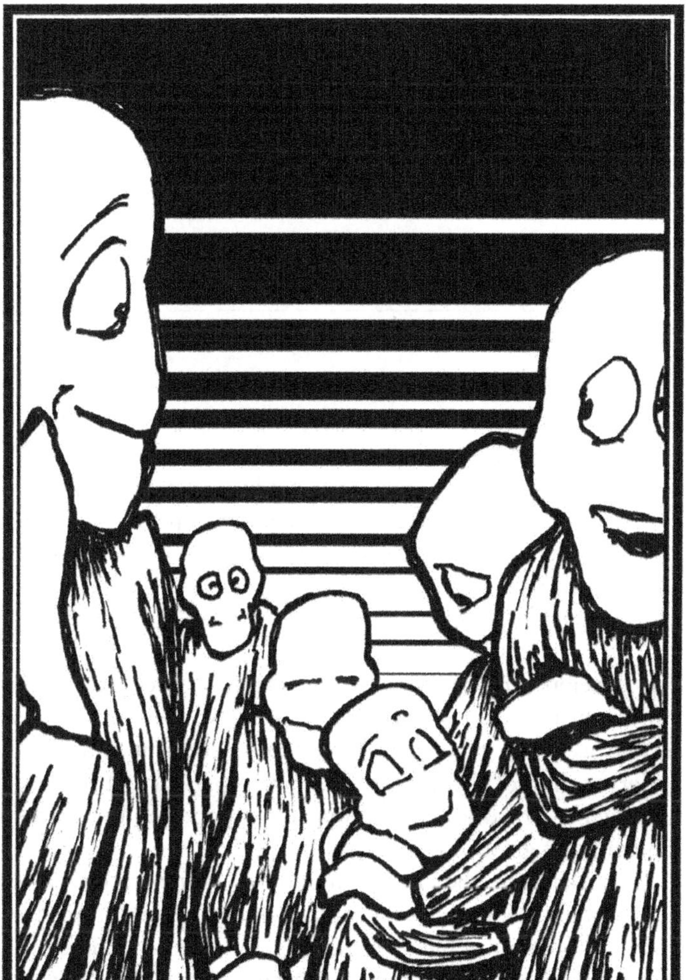

Feeling valued
for who we are.

Chapter 7
From a medical to a social model

> ... the social model refuses to see specific problems in isolation from the totality of disabling environments: hence the problem of unemployment does not just entail intervention in the social organisation of work and the operation of the labour market, but also in areas such as transport, education and culture.
>
> *Mike Oliver (1996, p.45)*

The development of the mental health service user/survivor movement has had many effects. As we have seen, it has helped service users to gain a different, more confident and positive understanding of themselves and their experience. It has begun to influence practitioners and impact on policy and practice. Its influence has grown to be international.

But perhaps the most important single result of the development of the survivors' movement is that it makes it possible to reframe mental health issues in new, different and more helpful ways. It offers the prospect of at last moving from a medical to a social approach to mental health issues. We have already touched more than once on the medical model in relation to mental health issues. This book has highlighted the continuing dominance of this model in the context of mental health and the mental health system. What can't be overstated is its pervasive and unhelpful nature, particularly in the experience of those on the receiving end.

The negative nature of the medical model

In a two-year national study, service users/survivors and others were asked how they thought mental health issues were understood in society (Beresford et al., 2010). The general consensus was that they were poorly understood and primarily associated with fear and danger. This appeared to originate from and be underpinned by a medicalised individual model of 'mental illness'. There was significant agreement that such a medicalised approach had few benefits to offer and was largely negative in effect.

Such a medical model was seen as all-pervasive in society. Professional approaches to mental health issues were also seen as being mainly medically based, seeing the problem as lying within the individual and responding primarily through the use of medication. Such professional interpretations were felt to have an important and unhelpful influence on public understandings. Among service users, the medical model was also seen as powerful; shaping, overshadowing and restricting their own understanding and attitudes.

Without acknowledging the dominance of the medical model in mental health, it is difficult to explain or understand the current over-reliance on 'treatment' with drug 'therapies' or the predominating focus in mental health research on trying to find new drugs to 'treat' 'mental illness' and its framing in terms of the diagnostic categories people are assigned to.

Participants in this study, in contrast, felt that a social approach to mental health issues brought with it a number of benefits (Beresford et al., 2010). It was likely to lead to better understanding, better personal support and a focus on the service user in provision, and could help change and improve wider attitudes by challenging narrow, medicalised understandings of mental health. Service users felt that more account needed to be taken of broader factors, to counter the individualisation of mental health issues. At the same time, there was a feeling among some mental health service users/survivors that it might be difficult for people to understand and implement a more social approach in a society strongly rooted in a medicalised individual model of mental illness.

A social model and mental health

There has long been some interest in and awareness of social issues in relation to mental health. But it has been marginalised by medical model approaches.

The traditional social approach

It may be argued that the emphasis here on the medical model in mental health overstates the issue; that there is a long and growing tradition of social approaches to and understandings of madness and distress, and that many psychiatrists and other clinicians are well aware of the role other, broader issues can play in people's lives and experience beyond their personal difficulties. After all, there has been a distinct field of social psychiatry and some progressive psychiatrists and psychologists have shown interest in social approaches. There is no question that there has been an awareness of social issues in some mental health disciplines and professions for some time. But this has tended to focus on social issues as factors in the creation of mental health problems. It has tended still to take mental illness or disorder as a given – to accept the idea – rather than attempt to reconceptualise mental health/wellbeing within a broader social framework. While mental health service users from my and my colleagues' study (Beresford et al., 2010) and other discussions seem to be supportive of a more social understanding of mental health issues, discussion of such a social approach in mental health has so far been relatively limited.

This is in sharp contrast to the disabled people's movement, where such discussions have been central to its development. The social approach that they have developed has been ground-breaking in its nature and implications. It has shaped the movement historically and internationally from its early days.

The importance of the social model of disability

The social model of disability was developed by the disabled people's movement. It has had a major impact on public policy and understanding in the UK and internationally, leading to major new legislation, new policies, new support roles and new approaches to service provision. It has challenged traditional Western understandings of disability. These were once entirely focused on the individual, seeing disability as located within the individual disabled person and resulting from some inherited or acquired impairment that restricted what they could do and could result in them being dependent and unable to live a 'normal' life. From the early 20th century, such individualised understandings of disability were overlaid by the medicalised thinking of emerging medical professions that appropriated disability as an area of expertise. The disabled people's movement saw this as resulting in a medicalised individual model of disability, which conceived of it as pathological and regarded disabled people as requiring segregation, institutionalisation, rehabilitation and welfare support (Oliver, 1996; Oliver & Barnes, 1998; Thomas, 2007).

The social model of disability that disabled activists developed instead drew a distinction between the physical, sensory or intellectual impairment or perceived impairment affecting an individual disabled person and the negative societal reaction to it. It is the latter that activists conceived of as disabling. Thus, disability was understood as a discriminatory and oppressive response to people seen as having an impairment, rather than a characteristic attached to the individual.

Discussion of the social model of disability among disability activists and in disability studies has been lively and fast-moving (Thomas, 2007). For disabled people, it has been a ground-breaking notion, shifting blame and responsibility for disability from the individual to the society and exploring the complex interrelations of the two. The social model of disability highlights the oppressive nature of the dominant social response to impairment, which excludes, segregates and stigmatises disabled people, creates barriers to their equality and participation, and discriminates against them, restricting their human and civil rights. This approach to understanding has encouraged disabled people to highlight the problems they face as primarily a civil rights (rather than welfare) issue. There is no doubt that the social model of disability has influenced public understanding of disability, as well as many disabled people's own perceptions of themselves.

The social model of disability is a radical shift in understanding because it does not just take account of social factors while retaining an essentially medical approach to disability. It also challenges such a medical approach because it takes account of the way that societal responses generate both understandings of disability and responses to it. It goes beyond the traditional 'nature versus nurture' approach to understanding people's situation as disabled people. It doesn't just rethink the meaning of 'disability'; it also prompts a radical rethink of its nature, causes, consequences and reduction.

The social model of disability helps us to understand:

- the many barriers disabled people still face in society. These include attitudinal, social, communication, economic, political and cultural barriers
- the discrimination that they face – the negative attitudes they encounter both from individuals and more broadly in society
- the oppressive way in which they can expect to be treated in society
- the way their human and civil rights tend to be restricted and undermined.

All these barriers and issues, of course, can also be seen to be experienced by mental health service users/survivors, just as disabled people have highlighted the barriers restricting them. Most participants in the study referred to above felt that they experienced barriers as mental health service users (Beresford et al., 2010). Thus the social model of disability offers a helpful starting point and framework for development in relation to the situation of mental health service users and madness and distress. It is easy to see how mental health service users are negatively affected by societal responses to them and the damaging effects these have. A social model of madness and distress is also likely to help us understand better:

- people's experience of madness and distress
- the societal barriers and discriminations operating in relation to madness and distress and their effects in disabling or 'maddening' people
- how some people's experience, perceptions and behaviour come to be seen as 'mentally ill'

- why some groups (particularly Black and minority ethnic people) face particular discrimination relating to madness and distress and the mental health system
- why madness and distress have also always been associated with and included people seen as non-conformist, resisting, disaffiliated and different.

The development of such a social model of madness and distress also coincides with a broader and growing interest in social approaches to mental health. This was signalled, for example, by the setting up of the Social Perspectives Network to explore and develop more social approaches to mental health and the publication of new books on the subject (Ramon & Williams, 2005; Tew, 2005). While some survivor activists have been working to develop these ideas, as my and colleagues' study found (Beresford et al., 2010), others less actively involved still seem to have concerns about an approach based on the social model of disability.

This reflects a similar situation with the initial development of the social model of disability itself, when many disabled people were wary or didn't understand it. Since then, disabled people have increasingly described it as providing a 'light-bulb' moment in their lives – a revelation that made it possible for them to challenge feelings of deficiency, guilt and blame and to think of themselves in new and positive ways. Far from being an abstract issue, it has a close bearing on people's ordinary day-to-day lives and understanding. The social model of disability does not seek to deny the individual experience of impairment, and nor does a social model of madness and distress ignore the distress that people may experience. Rather, the aim is to challenge the oppression and discrimination both groups face as a result and to develop more appropriate responses to their circumstances and experiences.

Just as the social model of disability has demonstrated its revolutionary potential for disabled people's lives, so we can expect that a comparable social model of madness and distress could have the same potential for service users/survivors. It offers the basis for a completely different way of coming at mental health issues – one that prioritises service users' perspectives and puts them and their lives in a wider context. It points to different ways for people to understand themselves and each other and different ways of addressing their experience and circumstances. It is to this that we turn next.

But first, we perhaps have to recognise that the social model of disability may not provide an adequate basis for this. This certainly seems to have been indicated by a further survivor-led study published in 2016 (Beresford et al., 2016). While this again highlighted survivors' concerns about traditional medical model understandings and their support for social approaches to mental health, it also revealed that survivors were divided in their support for the application of a social model of disability to issues of distress. Concerns ranged from the imposition of another label seen as negative – disabled – to a rejection of the assumption that their distress was necessarily appropriately conceived of as an impairment.

Chapter 8
Developing a new vision: Principles for the future

> My hope is for people to say, 'Do you know, 50 years ago, we used to say to people who'd been traumatised and abused and had terrible emotional problems, we used to say, "You're a schizophrenic or a manic depressive and you'll always be like that"'. We will look back and be horrified at the kind of things we do to one another today.
> *Jan Wallcraft, John Read & Angela Sweeney (2003, p.81)*

The focus in 'mental health' has often seemed backward-looking. Much energy, from both reformers and service users/survivors themselves, has been put into trying to improve the psychiatric system. Of course, there have been some improvements. Some service users/survivors have been able to access forms of support, particularly helpful 'talking therapies', that were not previously available to them. Some new drugs have been developed that, used sensitively, have improved the lives of some service users/survivors. Some practitioners really help through their understanding, commitment and kindness. There isn't quite the sense there once was that people who get caught up in the system become irretrievably lost in it.

However, it is difficult to feel that progress has matched that in other areas of medicine with which psychiatry might reasonably be compared. More often it feels like two steps forward and another step back, with constant cuts and changes, reductions in services, a continual emphasis on speeding up 'throughput' – for people to 'recover' and move on – and less time with support workers. As has been said, the psychiatric system seems to have an amazing capacity to resist progressive reform.

But, as we have seen, there is now a chance to start from a radically different paradigm. Service users/survivors and their organisations have developed their own ideas and values; their own theories and analysis; their own services and forms of support; their own arts and culture; their own forms of research and evaluation; their own literature and materials. In a relatively short time, they have challenged old assumptions, pioneered new approaches and influenced policy and practice for the better. But they have faced many obstacles and difficulties in taking forward their own proposals. And as they have made progress, these barriers seem to have grown.

Nonetheless, their own innovative ideas and developments provide a basis for a new service user-led social paradigm, based on a truly social approach to 'mental health' – or, as many survivors prefer to call it, madness and distress. A range of elements for such an approach can now be identified from existing experience. Most if not all of these elements already have a track record of development. However, what hasn't yet happened is for them to be put together as part of a properly supported strategic approach to 'mental health' policy and practice development and reform. They have yet to become central in mental health policy and practice so that they can be an everyday routine reality and choice for everyone who encounters the mental health system – whether as service provider or service user, or both.

The ideas and developments set out here build on the experience of many service users, as well as that of innovative policy makers, practitioners and managers. The values, principles and proposals offered here have been the subject of many people's thinking and many formal debates and informal discussions.

In this third part of the book, we look at what policy and provision in relation to madness and distress might look like if they were built on the understanding, knowledge and experience that is now available – particularly the emerging and developing ideas of service users – instead of being limited by our inheritance from the past. We begin with the kind of principles and values that such a new approach to madness and distress might be based upon.

The principles or values of such a socially based system are likely to include:

- prioritising self-advocacy
- being rights-based
- building on the philosophy of independent living
- self-management and self-support
- commitment to anti-oppressive practice
- supporting race equality and cultural diversity
- minimising compulsion
- breaking the bad/mad link
- prioritising participation
- equalising power relations.

We now look in more detail at each of these in turn before turning to the recent, ground-breaking development – Mad Studies.

Prioritising self-advocacy

At the heart of every movement, and this is as true for survivors as for any other group struggling against oppression and discrimination, is the need to be able to speak and act for yourself rather than have others speak for you. This is a fundamental starting point for regaining control of your life. It is a core principle for service user/survivor-led, rather than service system-led, ideas and understandings for making sense of madness and distress and changing the situation of mental health service users/survivors. This development has widely come to be called self-advocacy.

Advocacy more generally is essential in any system that seeks to safeguard service users' rights and can impose restrictions on these rights. With the extension of compulsory treatment into the community and the increasing number of service users/survivors who are becoming subject to sections (compulsory treatment under mental health legislation), the need for advocacy has become increasingly important. It was meant to be provided alongside the extension of compulsory 'treatment', but this has not been adequately developed. Advocacy, to be effective, needs to be:

- independent (of the service system)
- of good quality – employing skilled, trained and qualified advocates. There need to be recognised qualifications for advocates to ensure the provision of a high quality and reliable service
- available both on demand and without request. Not everyone knows about advocacy or the benefits it can offer. It is important that it is offered routinely and that, while it may of course be refused, it is always available. Without such independent advocacy, there can be no assumption that service users have been able to give their informed consent
- ongoing and available prior to a problem or a crisis. Advocacy, in practice, is often only available when something has gone seriously wrong or people's rights are being removed. All the evidence indicates that good advocacy is based upon the quality of relationship between advocate and service user. It is essential that people can have access to an advocate prior to problems developing
- equally available to Black and minority ethnic service users. There is a serious lack of Black and minority ethnic advocacy for and provided by Black and minority ethnic service users. Black and ethnic minority service users often value having Black and minority ethnic advocates and advocacy services, and this option needs to be readily available.

There are three other key requirements for good advocacy. First, it has to value service users' direct/lived experience. Many service users particularly value advocacy provided by people with shared understandings and experience. Advocacy policy should take this into account and support and encourage the recruitment and training of suitable candidates with experience as service users to offer such peer advocacy.

Second, advocacy should never be seen as an alternative to making services and processes as accessible, empowering and user-friendly as possible, so that any service user can negotiate them on their own. Third, and this is key, all forms of advocacy (legal, professional, peer and citizen advocacy) should primarily be directed to supporting self-advocacy – that is to say, it should promote the capacity of each individual service user to speak and act on their own behalf.

Being rights-based

Traditionally, responses to welfare service users like mental health service users/survivors and disabled people were based on definitions of their needs by outside 'experts'. First disabled people and then other groups felt that this created many problems and instead developed a rights-based approach, taking as the key yardstick for policy and practice how far it secured or undermined their civil and human rights. This included rights like:

- the right to freedom of movement
- the right to life
- the right to sexuality and reproduction
- freedom from want
- freedom from discrimination and to have effective redress against it
- to vote and participate in the political process
- the support that is needed to live your life on equal terms
- freedom of choice and opportunities
- the right to work
- freedom of information.

This is why the disabled people's movement campaigned for civil rights and freedom of information legislation. In the UK, reflecting international developments, such aspirations have now been taken forward to some extent by the extended provisions of UK disability discrimination legislation and the Disability Equality Duty, as well as the Human Rights Act and equalities legislation.

Many mental health service users/survivors are categorised as disabled people and have entitlements under the human rights, mental health and equalities legislation to disability benefits and to the direct payments and personal budget schemes pioneered by disabled people, which enable service users to shape their own package of support and, with the assistance they need, to control it themselves. A rights-based approach to mental health policy and practice highlights the importance of evaluating policy and provision in terms of the degree to which they support (or obstruct) service users' full and equal citizenship in society.

The philosophy of independent living

The idea of independent living is a simple but revolutionary one. It is a philosophy that was originally inspired by the disabled people's movement. It also works helpfully for people who use mental health services. It follows from the social model of disability. It is based on a belief that disabled people should be enabled to live their lives on as equal terms as possible alongside non-disabled people. It doesn't say how you should live or that you should live the same way as anyone else. Instead, it says you should have the same choice as anyone who isn't disabled (or who isn't a mental health service user), as far as possible. The philosophy of independent living turns traditional notions of independence on their head. It is not preoccupied with the individual or narrow ideas of personal autonomy. It does not mean 'standing on your own two feet or managing on your own'. Instead of seeing the service user as having a defect or deficiency requiring care, it highlights the need to ensure that they have the support they need to live their lives as fully as possible, on equal terms and interdependently with others (Morris, 1994). This support is not expected to come from unpaid family members or 'informal carers'.

The philosophy rejects the concept of care and replaces it with the idea of support. It sees independence as meaning being in a position to make your own decisions, rather than having to do everything for yourself (Campbell & Oliver, 1996; Morris, 2004). Instead of people being assessed on the basis of what they aren't able to do in order to qualify for 'care', under this model support is provided to enable them to live their lives as fully as possible in the way they wish. To sum up, there are two interrelated and key aspects to the philosophy of independent living. These are:

- ensuring people get the support that they need in order to live their lives as fully as they can, under their control, on as equal terms as possible with non-disabled people

- equalising their access to mainstream policy, services and amenities, like housing, health, education, employment and recreation.

This emphasises the relevance of independent living as a value base across public policy, as well as specifically in relation to human services. In England in 2008, departments across government signed up to these values in a national Independent Living Strategy (Office for Disability Issues, 2008). However, this initiative was ended by the national coalition government after 2010, and it needs to be said that public services are still a very long way from being organised and provided on a basis consistent with its now long-abandoned values.

You can see how this will also apply to people experiencing madness and distress. The aim should be to try to ensure that they can have the support they need to live as full and good a life as they can. It recognises that they may still face difficulties from their experience of distress but is based on trying to make sure that these can be minimised as far as possible and that lack of support is not made an additional problem for people.

Recovery

Independent living is not the only big 'new' idea that has developed in recent decades and has relevance to mental health issues and service users/survivors. Another is 'recovery'. This reflects the desire of service users and their movements to be recognised as active, contributing citizens. It has gained some support from service users. But, from its origins within the service user movement, it has been co-opted and shaped and advanced by state and service providers in ways that are completely contrary to the original intentions, and is widely regarded as ambiguous and contentious in its role and purpose. This may explain why there is no single agreed and consistent definition of recovery.

Nonetheless, the idea of recovery gained major interest in UK mental health policy and practice. There was talk of a 'recovery movement' and 'recovery colleges' were set up (Pilgrim, 2008). Many service users value the idea of recovery because it does not write them off as irreparably damaged or defective, but instead offers hope and the possibility of positive outcomes for their lives

(Turner-Crowson & Wallcraft, 2002). Other survivors, however, are highly critical of the concept's essentially medicalised basis and the associated emphasis on 're-ablement' and moving people into employment. While the philosophy of independent living developed by disabled people emphasises people's potentially continuing need for support to live their lives to the full, recovery instead implies that such support may become unnecessary and be withdrawn as people 'recover'. For this reason, some survivors see recovery as at least consistent with and in some cases supportive of the reactionary agenda of cuts, pressured integration into the labour market and increasing reliance on people's self-help and 'looking after themselves'.

Self-management and self-support

Service users have a central role to play in 'shaping their own lives'. Self-support and self-management have often been taken to mean a kind of 'self-help' approach, where the service user 'graduates' from formal support and manages on their own. This is often a bridge too far for service users and their loved ones and is actually experienced as withdrawal and being left to try to manage on their own.

There are more positive meanings for self-management and self-support that need to be developed instead. These are not concerned with trying to manage on your own, but with receiving and being in control of, as far as possible and desired, the support you need to manage your own life. Living as full and secure a life as possible on a sustainable basis can often also mean having support available at those times when you might again need it. This can be both formal and informal support. Just knowing the support can be available is sometimes enough in itself. The forms such support can take may include developing skills to maintain and run your own life, and playing the pivotal role (with support as needed) in running and negotiating the range of service interventions that might be needed in your life. The service user becomes the ringmaster rather than the passive bystander of what is happening in their life, and has an active role in determining:

- the nature and kind of support they receive
- any medication they receive

- the workers who work with them
- the particular service providers they access.

The service user is no longer the fly in the spider's web of services. Instead, they are the spider developing their own web of support and assistance, consistent with their own definitions of what they want and need. As has been said, to do this, they may also need capacity building or ongoing support in the form of advocacy, advice and information.

A more recent emphasis in health and social care policy discussions on 'personalisation' and 'personal budgets' chimes with ideas of self-management and self-support. The idea is that services should be shaped by and 'customised' to what each person needs, rather than people being fitted into a 'service-led' system. A key method for realising such personalisation has been seen as personal budgets, which offer people who are eligible a (real or notional) sum of money to spend on whatever support they would find most helpful. We look at this development in more detail in the next chapter.

Based on anti-oppressive practice

As we saw earlier, mental health policy and practice continue to be beset with problems of inequality and discrimination. The particular problems facing Black people and minority ethnic groups in the mental health system, as well as the difficulties facing women, particularly as mothers and in relation to safety, are well documented. A systematic approach in mental health practice to challenging discrimination based on difference on grounds of race, gender, sexuality, age, class, culture, faith, belief and disability is required. Such an approach has been developed in the fields of social work and social care practice. It will need to extend across occupational and professional groups and at all levels in the mental health system. It will need to be supported at organisational as well as individual levels.

Anti-oppressive practice needs to be linked with a systematic process of ongoing monitoring, evaluation, review and reward. Anti-oppressive practice does not generally sit comfortably with the restriction of people's rights, so the two concerns need to be considered in relation to each other. Service users and their organisations, rather than professionals, need to play a central role in shaping and developing anti-oppressive practice to ensure it meets their rights and needs (Wilson & Beresford, 2000).

Supporting race equality and cultural diversity

The mental health system has so far demonstrated a frequent failure to address issues of cultural diversity and race equality successfully. There can be little doubt that the system continues to be overshadowed by institutionalised racism. Black and minority ethnic service users (particularly some groups, like African-Caribbean young men and Irish people) have particularly negative experiences of the mental health system. As mentioned in the previous chapter, Black service users face disproportionately high risks of death in the system, of only being given drug 'treatments' and of over-prescription. While there is now a large and growing number of Black and minority ethnic practitioners, including psychiatrists and other professionals, psychiatry continues to be essentially Eurocentric in its orientation and operation.

Addressing issues of race equality and cultural diversity must be a priority for any new approach to mental health policy and practice. While there have been numerous government initiatives along these lines, so far they have not been successful. This commitment needs to be built into new social approaches to madness and distress. Black and minority ethnic service users and their organisations must be fully and effectively involved in efforts to reform the mental health system and to achieve the required commitment to race equality in its process, operation, capacity and goals.

In their definitive study of the survivor movement, Jan Wallcraft and her colleagues (2003, pp.31–42) highlighted both the discriminatory nature of the psychiatric system and how much more work is still needed for the survivor movement to be fully inclusive and proactive in addressing diversity. This includes tackling barriers and discriminations that operate in relation to all the equality issues including, of course, gender and sexuality issues as well as those of race equality. The issues raised by Wallcraft and colleagues continue to apply.

Minimising compulsion

Historically, almost invariably systems set up in response to madness and subsequently 'mental illness' have included strong elements of compulsion. Sometimes these have overshadowed and shaped the whole system, giving rise to the segregated and regulatory 'asylum' institutions established in the 19th century, where the overall regime was conditioned by concerns to secure, separate, morally educate, discipline and sometimes punish inmates. The concern of systems for the 'mad' and 'insane' to maintain social control has often spilled over into the imposition of punitive and abusive regimes. Such abusive regimes can be identified from the 15th century to the present.

Compulsion and the restriction of service users' rights continue to be aspects of increasing importance in current mental health systems. In England, forensic services and restrictions on people's rights have grown in scale rather than diminished. This has been underpinned and reinforced by current concerns about the risk posed by mental health service users. In the present political and media climate, there seems little likelihood of compulsion no longer being used in the psychiatric system. The immediate goal, however, must be to question and minimise it. The longer-term goal should be to end it. There are other ways of ensuring that people do not harm themselves or others than through the practice of forcible or compulsory 'treatment'.

The concept is a contradiction in terms. Alternatives include:

- providing rapid, appropriate and adequate support in response to people's requests to prevent them reaching crisis
- routine and effective use of (and adherence to requests set out in) crisis cards and advance directives
- the use of the provisions of the criminal justice system where people break the law and/or pose a threat to others
- ensuring the availability of valued and safe crisis, emergency and other provision for service users encountering serious difficulties.

Where service users' rights continue to be restricted, provisions need to be accompanied by adequate safeguards to ensure:

- immediate independent advocacy and support
- rapid processes of hearing and review
- rights to appeal and independent representation.

Breaking the bad/mad link

Since the policy shift from large institutions to 'care in the community', mental health service users have increasingly been associated by politicians and the right-wing media with violence, homicide, risk and threat to 'public safety'. While there is no evidence of any increase in violence or homicide from service users, this association has increasingly shaped policy responses and media presentations of mental health issues. It led to proposals for new legislation that generated unprecedented concerns about increased restrictions on the rights of mental health service users and widespread fears that many more service users would be drawn into the net of compulsion. Such legislation was then introduced – for example, to extend compulsory control into the community – and at least some of these fears have been justified. The lesson of numerous inquiries has been that homicides by mental health service users have tended to be linked with the failure of services to provide help when sought.

The assumed link between mental health service users and dangerousness has re-emerged to shape and dominate mental health policy, practice and thinking. It creates a damaging prospect for the many thousands of service users who pose no threat to anyone. It is likely to increase the stigma faced by service users and to make many reluctant to seek support from the mental health system.

However, there are more fundamental issues here that also need to be re-examined. First, it is hardly surprising that service users are associated with 'pathological' and deviant behaviour when their conceptualisation is based on a model of 'mental illness' that assumes pathology. Second, violence has increasingly been medicalised in Western societies like the UK on the basis of unevidenced assumptions that 'you must be mad to be so bad'. The medical model of mental illness is increasingly associated with violence. Thus, for example:

- common (physiological and psychological) responses to extreme threat and danger are reconceived as a form of mental disorder – 'post-traumatic stress disorder'
- 'mental disorder' is offered as an explanation for violence (including in US mass shootings) without reliable or consistent independent criteria or evidence to support it
- 'mental illness' and 'mental disorder' are routinely introduced as legal defences for criminal and violent behaviour
- committing violent acts without apparent remorse is identified as a form of 'severe and dangerous personality disorder'
- being subjected to sexual and other violent abuse or assault (especially in childhood) is offered as a sufficient predictor or explanation for an individual's own subsequent abusive or violent behaviour
- the perpetration of child sexual abuse is identified as a category of 'mental disorder'.

This requires fundamental reviews of:

- the concept of 'personality disorder' and 'borderline personality disorder'
- routine tendencies to associate 'mental illness' with violence, without reliable independent evidence
- the common use of 'mental disorder' as a defence for violent and sexual attacks and abuse in order to avoid or mitigate custodial sentences.

Prioritising participation

User involvement, empowerment and partnership have all become 'buzz words' in mental health. Yet still in wider society, mental health service users face some of the most serious problems of exclusion, stigma and powerlessness. While efforts have been made to increase the involvement of service users in mental health services, their position and status in society are still largely marginal.

Prioritising the participation of mental health service users/survivors offers an effective basis for challenging this situation.

Instead of seeing participation as merely an add-on component to service provision, it needs to become a central concern for policy in the widest sense. Existing government requirements for the participation and partnership of mental health service users can provide an effective lever to help achieve this. Participation needs to be recognised as both a central concern in the process and as a key purpose of policy, provision and practice. In this way, participation can provide a central means by which service users can:

- exert influence over their experience of and negotiations with the mental health system
- influence decision-making processes in the mental health system and other policies and services impacting on their lives.

It should also be developed as a priority goal, to ensure that mental health service users have the greatest possible opportunities to participate fully in all aspects of society according to their wishes and abilities – for example, in education, employment, recreation, networks, social and family life and in their communities.

In Chapter 10, we discuss 'user-controlled organisations'. These offer a key route to effective participation in every sense.

Equalising power relations

Experience of madness and distress is often, but not always, a disempowering phenomenon. Frequently, however, experience of the mental health system adds to rather than reduces this sense of powerlessness. As we have seen, it becomes another problem to be dealt with, rather than feeling like part of a solution. If mental health services are to support people's wellbeing and act as a positive rather than negative experience, a help rather than a burden, then they need to be a positive in people's lives. If they are to achieve that, then they will need to be based on a fundamental commitment to equalise relationships within them. This can be seen as a key problem in existing services, which helps to explain the frequent problems of abuse, violence and poor conditions that service users report. Mental health services have frequently tended to be institutionalised, and all the evidence is that such institutionalised services have the most difficulty ensuring and maintaining equal power relationships. The tendency in current services may be towards inequality because of existing inequalities of power, status and credibility between service users, providers and professionals, but these can be challenged. Their operation must be regularly and routinely audited at all levels to establish how much this happens and to stop it continuing.

There are also other ways of ensuring that people can work in more equal and collaborative ways, which have been developed in other fields and where there have also been some pioneering initiatives in mental health provision.

These include:

- increasing the involvement of people with experience as service users as trainers and educators in professional and occupational training and education
- encouraging the recruitment of people with service-user experience and appropriate skills into the mainstream mental health workforce
- rewarding workers for working in more participatory and inclusive ways as part of qualification requirements, performance review and promotion processes
- developing de-institutionalised approaches to support and services that provide 'open' rather than closed regimes, so as to encourage services, service workers and users to be in more routine contact with the wider world.

All of these will build understanding and challenge disempowering barriers between mental health services and those they are intended to support.

Mad Studies

Finally in this chapter, we come on to one of the most significant, positive and potentially ground-breaking developments that have taken place between the writing of the first and this edition of this book. Amid all the negatives we have had to report here – the continuing cuts in public services in the industrialised West, the rise in global poverty and inequality, and the pressures on our physical and mental wellbeing from years of neoliberal ideology, without apparent end in sight – a new development, building on the foundations laid by the collective survivor past, has emerged.

This is Mad Studies. Mad Studies has the potential to pull together all the positive ideas and developments that have been discussed in this chapter. Moreover, for the first time, it provides a route to fill the philosophical gap that has often seemed to characterise survivor activism: the lack of a core, shared philosophy that recognises the rights, needs and values of those of us facing madness and distress. Such a philosophy could provide a route out of the many difficulties, misrepresentations and misunderstandings that we have long faced.

In a relatively short space of time, Mad Studies has become an international movement. It first emerged in Canada and its rise is particularly associated with the publication of a book, *Mad Matters*, in 2013, that brought together that experience and the ideas that grew out of it and made it available to an international audience (LeFrançois et al., 2013). Mad Studies is both an area of intellectual development and a movement – it is a praxis that combines action and thought.

Four core values shape Mad Studies as it is currently defined. These are:

- it is ideologically positioned
- it is based on collectivity
- it builds on alliances
- it values lived experience as a basis for knowledge.

While Mad Studies has emerged in the 21st century as a pioneering innovative development, it is also directly linked to principles and values from the survivor movement's earliest days, including, for example, the work of pioneering survivor activists like Peter Sedgwick. So Mad Studies represents less a changed direction of travel for survivor action and more a reaffirmation and clarification of founding principles. The three defining characteristics of Mad Studies are:

1. It rejects a traditional biomedical model and the theoretical and treatment assumptions tied to it. It values and draws

instead on a wide range of other understandings, including those from feminist, disability and queer studies, rejecting medical dominance. It prioritises social understandings and interpretations, as did the disabled people's movement before it.

2. It values and places an emphasis on first-person or experiential knowledge, based on the belief that survivors' experience, lives, viewpoints and knowledge must be accorded equal status with professional knowledge and expertise. At the same time, it gives value to the first-person knowledge of everyone, not just those who are psychiatrised, acknowledging the complexity of our identities and all that each of us experiences and can bring to bear.
3. Because Mad Studies has a place for all our first-hand experiential knowledge, it makes it possible for a wide range of roles and standpoints to contribute equally to the discipline – if they accept its core principles. It isn't only we survivors/mental health service users who can be part of Mad Studies on this basis; so can its allies, professionals, researchers, loved ones, and so on, as long as they are prepared to sign up to its core principles (Beresford & Russo, 2022).

Mad Studies has gained massive interest and has also been closely critiqued by both survivor and non-survivor commentators. It has particularly come in for criticism for its potential exclusions. The main concerns have been its potential to be elitist, academicised, racialised and tied to the Global North at the expense of the Global South; that it inadequately addresses diversity and that it is based on exclusionary language. Another concern is that, following in the footsteps of the old anti-psychiatry movement and early survivor activism, it is narrowly focused on opposing psychiatry. This would be particularly unhelpful if it is to be seen as having a global relevance, given that psychiatry is much more marginal in many Global South countries. The fact that these objections have been raised so early in its development can also be seen as a potential strength, as it has been encouraged to acknowledge and overcome them. Certainly, such discussion figures large in its rapidly growing literature and debates.

Chapter 9
Developing a new vision: Survivor-led approaches to support

> Patient-controlled services: A real alternative to the institutions that destroy the confident independence of so many.
> *Judi Chamberlin (1988, front cover)*

In the last chapter we looked at the kinds of principles and values that follow from a survivor-led and social approach to madness and distress. We now consider the sort of support and provision that the evidence from and experience of service users/survivors and their organisations suggest is likely to be helpful for the future as the basis for improving the control they have over their lives and the quality of their support. If the old system has often seemed preoccupied with controlling and individualising people, then, as the US survivor pioneer Judi Chamberlin said, for the future, 'liberation is the goal' and it is most likely to be achieved through our own efforts as mental health service users/survivors (Chamberlin, 1988, p.xiii).

The elements that will go to make up the practice and provision of such an alternative approach to madness and distress are likely to include:

- self-definition of needs
- user-controlled and self-run services
- peer support

- valuing holistic and complementary approaches
- user-led training and education
- self-run schemes for personal support
- encouraging community development approaches
- the development of new roles and new approaches.

All of these are about ensuring people get the kind of support that they need to live their lives as well as they can and to be in a position to make informed judgements and decisions about what will most help. Taken together, they make it possible for as many people as possible to be included in and benefit from such a new, holistic approach to support. At the heart of them all lies the idea and achievement of user-controlled or self-run services, so particular attention is paid to these here. But the story starts with people being given the chance to work out what they want and what would most help them.

Self-definition of needs

At present, people mainly go to services and services offer what they are used to providing or what they think service users need. We know that this doesn't work well. But equally, just being told that you can make choices and have what you want doesn't necessarily mean much if you have low expectations, little idea or information about what might be possible and have spent years in disempowering and institutionalising situations. People need first to be in a position to make meaningful choices.

People's human and civil rights, and safeguarding them, need to be central in a reformed approach to mental health – or, as I would prefer to describe it here, 'madness and distress'. The mental health system has traditionally been based on ideas of 'need'. This approach has tended to have a number of shortcomings. As we have seen, it has generally been based on the definitions and judgements of policymakers, professionals and organisations, using an individualistic medicalised model. This approach has emphasised people's inabilities and deficiencies, rather than their capacities – what they can't do rather than what, with support, they might be able to do. In order to qualify for support, people have had to demonstrate their deficiencies. This has worked against preventive approaches to madness and distress. It frequently means that people cannot access a small amount of support to enable them to maintain their lives and activities, which then puts these in jeopardy. It has also been a destructive approach to welfare benefits policy.

As Judi Chamberlin said many years ago, 'The definition of need would come from the client' (1988, p.18). It is important to move to a model based on self-definition of needs where, with appropriate advocacy, information and support, service users are able to identify the necessary support to enable them to do the things they would like to do. This was the ostensible aspiration at the heart of the UK care management and care programme approach introduced in 1993 with the Community Care reforms.

To work, this requires:

- independent, reliable and accessible information
- independent advocacy, including peer advocacy and support for self-advocacy
- independent (non-medicalised) assessment.

Disabled people's organisations initially made some progress in developing such roles, training and accreditation, enabling service users to provide such support on an independent basis, informed by shared experience. So there is knowledge to turn to. Survivor-led organisations similarly have pioneered such activities. In this way, service users who need and want support are much more likely to come to the starting line knowing what they want and confident enough to be assertive in getting it. We have learned much from all this insight and innovation. But still it has largely remained at the edge of policy, rather than centrally informing and transforming it. This tells us more about the inflexibility of 'mental health' (and, indeed, disability) policy than about the lack of energy for user-led reform. We have to be aware of these barriers if we are to deal with them, but we should not allow them to discourage us from the paths we need to take. I know that is easier said than done; I speak as someone who has tried to keep going! Whenever user-led approaches have been supported and evaluated, they have shown their merits and how much they are valued by their service users.

User-controlled and self-run services

At the heart of a radically altered support system for people with experience of madness and distress and the psychiatric system are self-run or user-controlled services. They are absolutely key to transforming mental health policy and practice and the lives of mental health service users/survivors.

There is now a long track record of mental health service users/survivors pioneering their own user-controlled services. Judi Chamberlin was writing about 'patient-controlled services' in her ground-breaking book *On Our Own* (1988), first published in 1978. This can be seen as part of a broader development of user-controlled services developed by service users and disabled people. This now has a history of many years' innovation. These facilities include safe houses and crisis houses, drop-in and day centres, helplines, advocacy and peer-support schemes and employment opportunities, residential, housing, employment and training projects and environmental and gardening schemes.

In the mental health field, user-controlled services have tended to break out of the narrow, medicalised approach to responding to mental health problems and instead frame support in broader social terms that address the wider problems and barriers that service users highlight. They have been organised as cooperatives, social enterprise schemes and charitable organisations. They can be, as Judi Chamberlin highlighted, a network of provision and support, flexible so that people can move within it as they need more or less or different kinds of support (1988, p.18). This has been an international development, even if, as we have already noted, it has often been held back or undermined by traditional policy and services. Such user-led services have been run and managed by service users with service-user workers.

We also have reliable evidence about such user-controlled services. A major national study supported by the Big Lottery (Barnes & Mercer, 2006) explored the views of all stakeholders involved with such services, from the service-user trustees responsible for their governance, the managers and the user practitioners providing them, to (crucially) the service users who accessed them. The results were overwhelmingly positive. Service users valued such services, felt that they were more supportive

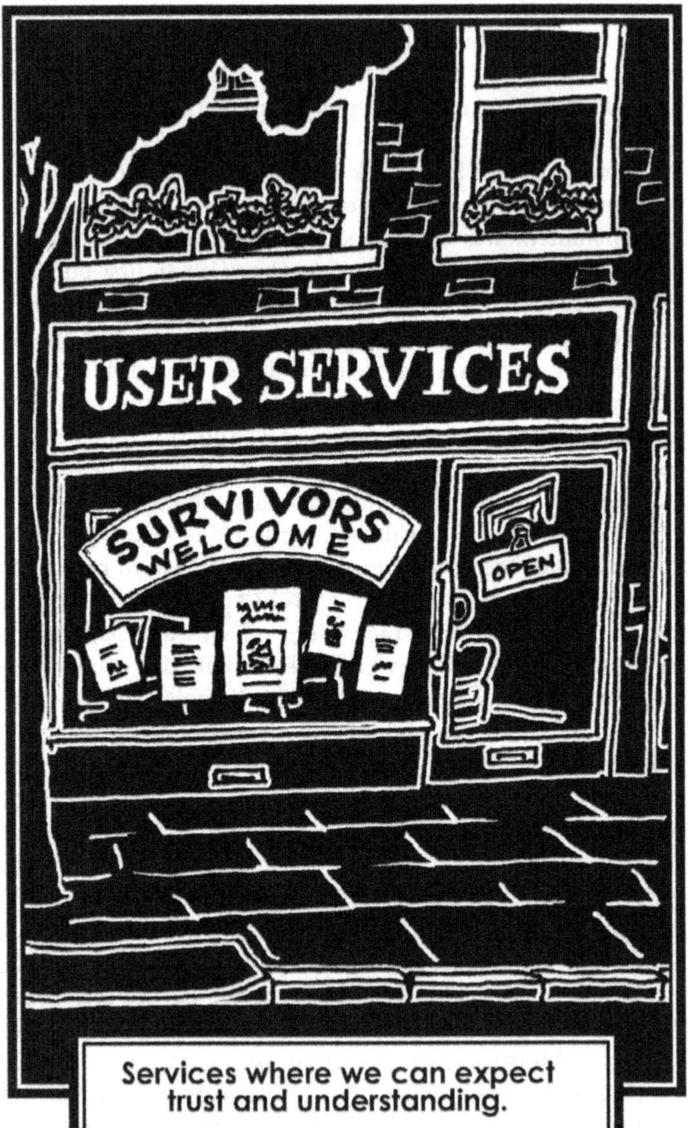

Services where we can expect trust and understanding.

and sensitive than other traditional arrangements and highlighted their benefits. Such services were particularly popular among service users and improved their quality of life. This has important economic and social benefits for the service user, their family and the local community.

Judi Chamberlin's inspiring work is still invaluable for understanding the ground-breaking role of user-controlled services. She based it on the US experience, while also looking at developments in other countries. Her experience connects closely with that in the UK. As she wrote:

> Patient-controlled alternatives can provide services to people without the demoralising consequences of the authoritarian, hierarchical structures of traditional mental health services. When the emphasis is on people helping one another, the gulf between 'patient' and 'staff' disappears. Someone can seek help from others without being thought of as sick or helpless. (Chamberlin, 1988, p.6)

She also wrote:

> Non-professional, client-controlled services don't divide people into 'sick' and 'well', 'helper' and 'helped'. They see every person as having a combination of strengths and weaknesses, and the need for help in one area does not negate the ability to help others also. (Chamberlin, 1988, p.68)

Judi Chamberlin warned against services that presented themselves as 'user-controlled' where service users were employed to do the work or did it as volunteers but control stayed with traditional mental health professionals.

She was suspicious of 'alternative' services based on 'partnership' or collaboration models with professionals, believing that the latter tend always to take over. She argued instead for a separatist model where 'ex-patients provide support for one another and run the service… they provide a real alternative to the dehumanising effects of mental health 'care' (Chamberlin, 1988, p.94):

> On the other hand, the alternatives built on the supportive and separatist models – the true alternatives – have been designed by ex-patients who are not merely passive recipients of a service but who are actively involved in running it… In the professional versions of alternatives… the professional is always the senior partner. (1988, p.106)

Tina Coldham, when Chair of the National Survivor User Network and writing to me as a long-term activist, made similar points from a UK perspective:

> To some, user-led services might seem like the lunatics running the asylum. However, mad people are moved to provide user-led provision for their peers for very good reasons. Firstly, we can have enormous insight into our distress and develop incredible empathy towards others as a result of this. Secondly, because we are grounded in our experiences, users can be very objective and committed to making what matters work. More so, we harbour a deeper understanding of what matters and therefore are driven by a passion for getting it right, particularly when we feel others miss the point. User involvement is a means to an end; that end is people being able to get on with their lives mentally well. However, involvement often becomes a whole industry with a purpose of its own, and doesn't actually impact upon people's lives as the end product.
>
> Users and survivors are brave to challenge the vast mental health system from within. Some of us are running alternatives to this as a way of challenging the status quo in a positive manner that can have real impact upon people's lives. We can be 'madly' creative and innovative in developing solutions to our problems, and in doing so, inspire others, and develop user leadership. I was once told, 'If you want commitment, get people who have been committed!' What more can I say? (Personal communication)

Service users and their organisations have found it very difficult to get the funding and other support to develop their own services on any scale. Their status has often been precarious, and valued services have had to close through failure to secure funding. Service users are thus frequently denied this choice, and even where such services are available, mainstream services are sometimes unaware of their existence and don't refer service users to them.

Over a number of years now, successive UK governments have argued for the importance of services being available from a wide range of providers. They have highlighted the problems they associate with the state dominating the provision of services. They have frequently called for an expanded role for the voluntary sector. There has been a massive expansion in private sector provision, which has become the major provider of social care services. This pressure for a move away from state provision is closely in tune with the development of service user-controlled services. Yet the irony is that, over this period, such services still remain marginal, both in mental health and in wider health and social care provision. This is not for want of service users trying. Service users and their organisations have worked hard to expand the kind of non-medicalised provision that they have shown a particular capacity to provide successfully. However, they have continued to face big barriers. As Colin Barnes, Emeritus Professor at the Centre for Disability Studies at Leeds University, said of the pioneering developments of disabled people:

> In spite of entrenched opposition from established service providers, services such as Disability Information and Advice Lines (DIAL), peer counselling and support facilities, integrated accessible housing schemes for disabled and non-disabled people, direct payment schemes for personal assistance and technical aids and equipment, were all pioneered and provided by grass roots CIL-type [Centres for Independent Living] groups during the 1970s and 80s. (Personal communication)

User-controlled services have received little support or encouragement in local or national commissioning policies, for all their rhetoric of challenging traditional patterns of service provision and the 'monopoly' of state provision. The typical pattern of provision is still based on large for-profit organisations and traditional big charities, purchased through block commissioning for economies of scale, standardised for large numbers of people. This advantages the lowest bidders, who also tend to employ workers at the lowest rates and with the poorest conditions.

The same obstacles in the way of user-controlled services that Judi Chamberlin identified more than 40 years ago still apply. It is difficult to secure funding, professionals are often opposed to them, and service users may be lacking in confidence and capacity. While there have been outstanding examples of innovation from user-controlled services, these have tended to be insecure and have often been short-lived, for want of wider official support. The insecurity and under-funding of such services means that their skilled and experienced user-workers often have to move on to conventional services, to ensure some job security in their own lives. Often the aspirations to provide truly user-controlled services have been subverted because service users haven't been granted the status or credibility to take them forward and more traditional organisations have taken over such initiatives and ideas, undermining their user-controlled principles in the process.

As well as stifling their development and security by restricting their funding, such survivor-led developments have also been compromised by being subverted by the dominant psychiatric system. That is to say, while ostensibly being advanced, often they are reframed in terms of the values, understandings and philosophy of prevailing arrangements. Most significantly, what this means is that they are recast in psychiatric terms. We have also seen peer and lived-experience roles reduced to ancillary ones, without clear career development, side-lining those who take them on and imposing a glass ceiling on them. This has been reported internationally by survivor activists and researchers.

We might have hoped that there would be growing opportunities for user-controlled services through the expansion of personal budgets and self-directed support schemes, which I discuss in more detail in this chapter. They offer people the chance to choose their own 'package of support' and we might expect many people to opt for user-controlled support. In 2012, we asked whether governments would support this wholeheartedly and hoped that service users/survivors and our organisations might make a difference by making our voices heard loud and clear. However, the determined thrust of policy as a result of Conservative governments in the UK and neoliberal ideology more generally has seriously restricted progress.

A strategic approach to supporting the development of user-controlled and self-run services is key for a different future. This will need the allocation of specific, secure funding to kick-start such provision. Such services also offer important employment, training and career opportunities for mental health service users/survivors. More support and evaluation will be needed to maximise these opportunities and to enhance skill development and career opportunities for service users. They offer a ground-breaking and unique way in which 'the helped' can be helpers and the helping helped. So far, however, no major UK political party has pledged its support for such an approach to mental health policy.

Peer support

We have already touched on peer support – arrangements of different kinds where people can draw on their lived experience to help others in similar positions. There are many approaches to peer support. These can be more and less formal. Service users/survivors have long highlighted the value they get from the support that they can offer each other because of the shared understandings and experience that provide a key basis for trust-building and mutuality. Some service users develop 'mentoring' relationships with others to provide guidance and support. Others have formed counselling relationships with each other based on friendship and shared experience.

For example, a long-term mental health service user described to me an arrangement that he and a couple of survivors had used over several years. Initially it was a support group where they would meet, and then it became a virtual support group where they did not physically meet. They would begin by taking turns talking about their situation without interruption for about five minutes, only occasionally giving feedback to each other. People were listened to and found it really helpful to talk about what was happening to them in an atmosphere of non-judgement and understanding.

It is also worth quoting Anne Wilson (the pseudonym of a mental health service user/survivor) at length about the positives she has gained from 'co-counselling':

> I was a mental health service user and was well and truly caught up in the psychiatric system. I met someone who was involved in co-counselling and was really interested in what she told me. When I told the mental health professionals working with me that I wanted to try co-counselling, all of them advised against it because they said people like me (with 'schizophrenia') 'needed trained mental health professionals, not amateurs'.
>
> Seven years later, I picked up the phone and dialled the number in an advert for a CCI (Co-Counselling International[1]) 'fundamentals' course. The person who answered the phone wasn't at all fazed by my saying that I'd had psychiatric treatment in the past (I had by then taken myself off medication and because I'd moved around the country several times, the mental health professionals had lost track of me). She did say that, in order to do co-counselling, I would need to have the emotional resources to listen to and support another person, which I felt I did, so I joined the course.
>
> Doing co-counselling fundamentals training has to be the best thing I have ever done in my life, but probably not for the reason you think!
>
> Co-counsellors work in pairs and, halfway through, 'client' and 'counsellor' swap places so you each spend an equal amount of time as both client and counsellor. It is therefore a relationship of equals and there is no possibility of an 'expert' or 'professional' telling you what is 'wrong with you', as when it is your turn to be the client, you are in charge. This was a revelation, but nothing like as much of a revelation as the most important thing for me about co-counselling, which was hearing other people talk about their experiences and concerns when they were the client and I was the counsellor. What I realised was that a lot of

1. www.co-counselling.org.uk

> the 'symptoms' and strange perceptions I experienced (which psychiatrists had attributed to 'schizophrenia' in my case) were in fact quite common experiences – I realised this because I co-counselled with many, many people who, during the course of their co-counselling sessions, spoke about being in stressful situations and experiencing some of what I experienced, maybe in not such an extreme way or over such extended periods, but nevertheless very similar experiences to my own. I can't tell you what they said as the content of co-counselling sessions is strictly confidential, and confidentiality is something which co-counsellors take very seriously.
>
> Through co-counselling therefore I came to see myself as a 'normal' person. This was a fantastic achievement, given all the negative and damning roles I'd been assigned by the psychiatrists – roles which I had also deeply internalised. And I also made many friends.
>
> That's not to say however that co-counselling has been a bed of roses, for (just as in the population at large) there are some co-counsellors who hold 'mentalist' attitudes. For me, the best co-counsellors have been people who have also had encounters with psychiatry themselves. Being involved in CCI has also enabled me to develop friendship networks locally, nationally and internationally. (Personal communication)

More generally, peer support, as we have already heard, is one of the areas of user involvement and survivor employment that has been most undermined and corrupted by existing psychiatric services internationally, with peer support workers writing at length about the way their insights and contribution are abused and misused – reshaped to fit psychiatry, rather than vice versa.

The particular circumstances created by the Covid-19 pandemic have also highlighted the value of different and new ways of working, many of which play to the strengths and circumstances of people experiencing distress and/or mental health services users. They show that virtual/distanced working – which many service users have argued for and found more accessible – can and does work and can play to their particular circumstances and difficulties. We don't have to be in a room

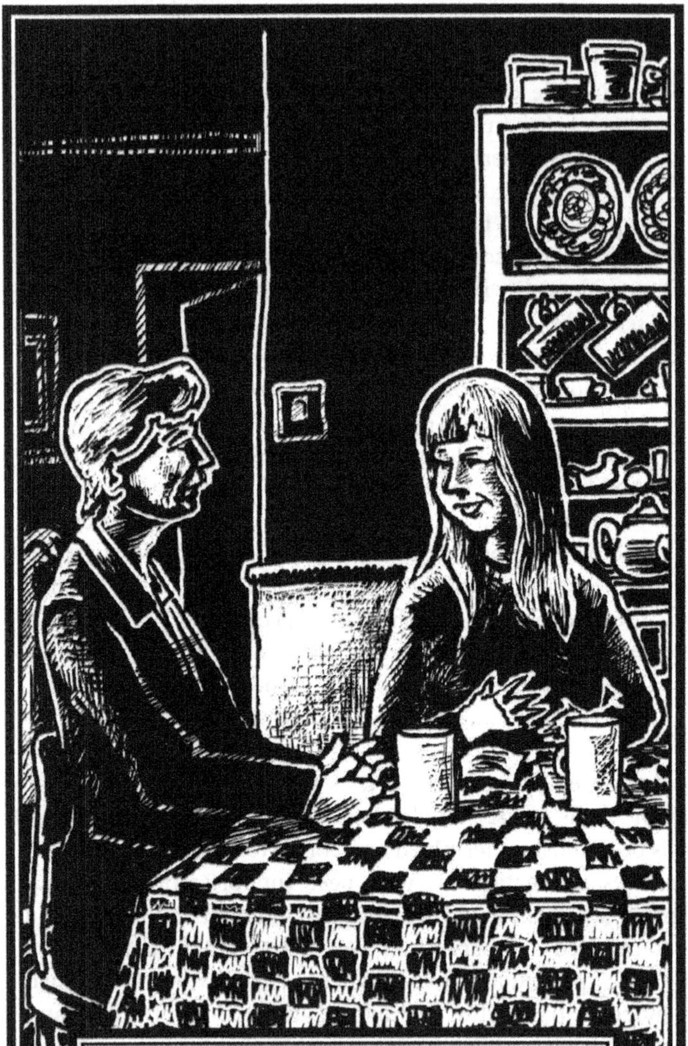

Where the helper is
also the helped.

together to help or be helped. What's really needed is a meld of the best of both the traditional and post-pandemic approaches – face-to-face and virtual/distanced helping. For some mental health service users and others experiencing madness and distress, who feel confident with computers and have online access, this can be a real route to improved access, involvement and support. But of course, for many others, the barriers, exclusions and digital divide would have to be overcome first if online arrangements were to be truly inclusive and anti-discriminatory (Williams et al., 2021).

Valuing holistic and complementary approaches

The medical base of mental health policy and thinking – the tendency to separate the mind from the body – has encouraged the prevailing medicalised 'treatment' responses to people included as mental health service users. This has been reinforced by the bureaucratic tendency to organise and compartmentalise according to policy and administrative concerns, rather than on the basis of individual lives, rights, wants and needs.

When the UK government made an attempt to move away from the dominance of drug therapy to introduce more 'talking therapies', it seemed to do this in a similarly mechanistic way. The Improving Access to Psychological Therapies programme (IAPT, now renamed NHS Talking Therapies) placed a strong emphasis on cognitive behavioural therapy (CBT) rather than the wider range of such therapies, offered only a limited number of one-to-one sessions, and employed practitioners with a narrow range of skills and experience to provide initial guided self-help before access to an experienced therapist could be achieved. Service users/survivors voiced concerns that these sessions just raised issues for them without further support being available for them to deal with these issues.

Traditional 'scientific' prejudices also discouraged the development and application of the wide range of complementary therapies available. The latter have also come in for criticism because they are rarely subjected to the randomised control trials (RCTs) that are the current 'gold standard' test for effectiveness for any approaches that are adopted in the NHS. Thus, such approaches to support are still treated with suspicion in the mainstream, although this has begun to change. User-led and voluntary organisations, as well as private practitioners, are increasingly offering them. They are also entering mainstream statutory services. But they are far from being a routine option for many service users, and especially not for the majority on low income who cannot afford to pay a private practitioner.

Yet such services are particularly suited and receptive to a holistic approach to emotional and mental distress. Policy and provision need to develop a more holistic approach to the rights and needs of service users. This includes:

- seeing the individual as a person, not a collection of problems, symptoms or deficits
- integrating policies so as to recognise the interrelation of different aspects of the person's life and connect policies across traditional sector silos to meet these needs. It is not enough to see policy and provision for mental health service users as the sole concern of the NHS or social care. The wide range of relevant policy areas, including income, public transport, leisure and recreation, education, training and employment, must also be taken into account and audited against the inclusive and participatory goals of the mental health system
- giving equal recognition to complementary approaches to healing that are valued by service users, and accepting a wider range of ways to evaluate their effectiveness and acceptability.

User-led training and education

Service users, their organisations, progressive practitioners and service organisations have long argued that involving service users in staff and professional education and training can play a crucial role in improving service cultures and making them more 'user-centred'. Even on a piecemeal basis, the introduction of 'user training', the development of a growing number of user trainers and the introduction of 'training for user trainers' have all made a valuable impact on mental health provision and practice. What is still needed is a coherent and systematic approach to user involvement in mental health training that goes much further than tokenistic invitations to service users to offer one-off sessions on their personal experience.

The three-year BA social work qualification introduced in 2003 required service user and carer involvement in all aspects of professional education. Central funding was also made available to operationalise it. There is now similar provision in all social work qualifying courses, including the more recent fast-track ones. It is such a coherent approach (without funding support, sadly), that has also been developed in allied health qualifications. It is needed across all mental health occupations, professions and disciplines. It is greatly valued by social work students and educators on such courses. This type of approach needs to include user involvement in recruitment, curriculum development, teaching, assessment and accreditation. It should draw fully on materials produced by mental health service users and their organisations, to complement learning materials from other sources. These are now increasingly available.

Self-run schemes for personal support

The main way in which the disabled people's movement in the UK was able to advance the idea of 'independent living' based on a social model of disability was through the introduction of 'direct payments' or 'self-run personal assistance' schemes. What these mean essentially is that the individual service user, after assessment, receives an allocation of state funding directly, with which they are then able to purchase the 'package of support' that they want, to meet their support needs as they define them.

Disabled people have often used this money to directly employ 'personal assistants' to meet their support requirements. So far, such direct payments schemes, which were subsequently extended by legislation to become a mandatory option for a wider range of service users, including many mental health service users, have represented the strongest expression of 'user-controlled' support for health and social care service users.

Since then, much more emphasis has been placed on such schemes by policymakers and politicians under the heading of 'personalisation', in the form of personal and individual budgets and 'self-directed support' schemes, in both social care and health services. They can provide marvellous opportunities for mental health service users to get the social support that the traditional mental health system has so often failed to provide.

However, that seems to have been less and less the case as funding for public services has been reduced and social care in England has become more crisis-ridden and problematic. Major obstacles in the way of this happening have increasingly emerged. First, the level of funding provided is now far more likely to be based on what limited money is available, rather than what support people actually need to live their lives to the best, in line with the philosophy of independent living. Second, service users have often not had the degree of support needed to make such schemes work and become accessible to many, so that only a small proportion of people have had the confidence to access them. Third, particularly in relation to mental health service users, restrictions are often placed on what kind of support people are allowed to purchase because of assumptions either that they are not sufficiently responsible or that there might be a media backlash to the kind of support services they find helpful.

Thus, so far, a relatively small number of mental health service users are accessing direct payments and personal budgets, although the schemes rapidly gained support and interest from mental health service users. They made it possible for service users to reassess their support needs in non-medicalised terms and secure the kind of assistance that they find helpful. This includes personal assistance, out of hours help, help with day-to-day tasks (like cooking, going out and shopping), and counselling, advice and 'talking therapies'. Some service users initially were also able to pool parts of their budgets to buy things as a group, like training, equipment and recreational opportunities.

More often, though, personalisation has meant little more than local authorities adding up the cost of conventional services being made available and then calling this notional sum a 'managed budget', with nothing actually changing for the individual service user.

Self-run personal assistance schemes are not a panacea and they should be seen as an option, rather than the only approach available to service users. However, where properly implemented, survivors receiving them have reported fewer inpatient hospital stays and the possibility of avoiding crises through having support in advance of their situation worsening (Newbigging & Lowe, 2005).

If such schemes are to work for the wide range of mental health service users who are now entitled to them, then experience strongly indicates that local user-controlled organisations need to be established and properly funded and supported to offer back-up, financial and technical support and advice so that every service user (regardless of their experience and expertise) is able to take advantage of them without it being burdensome or difficult, even if they are in crisis or going through a particularly bad time. The evidence from direct payments schemes for disabled people also highlights that the health of people receiving these schemes tends to improve and that they gain transferable skills that help them return to employment if they so wish (Beresford & Slasberg, 2023). The effects such schemes can have for people are summed up by Andy Smith, a mental health service user and strong advocate for their transformative benefits:

> In many respects people like me are the most persuasive argument in favour of self-directed support. Having used the funds to liberate myself and gain control and independence, the logical next step was to get myself educated to a level that would permit me to attempt to similarly improve the lives of other service users. Since my involvement with SDS [self-directed support] both my leisure and career options have multiplied. If it worked for me, it might work for you. (Personal communication)

Unfortunately, the more general picture across the board has been of personal budgets being reduced in value, not meeting the full support needs of service users and often leaving them at the mercy of the additional employer risks and responsibilities and insurance issues that they incur, without adequate information, support or safeguards.

Encouraging community development approaches

Mental health policy and provision have generally tended to operate in relation to the individual. However, initiatives that seek to enable people to come together to achieve change and support have a long and successful track record in this field. These include, for example, the pioneering work of truly democratic therapeutic communities that offer peer-group support, as well as group work and group therapy. Community development approaches, therefore, are likely to have a particular contribution to offer in social approaches to madness and distress. They make it possible to:

- reach out and involve a diverse range of service users, rather than expecting people to come forward themselves
- challenge isolation by operating proactively rather than reactively
- engage with and understand service users in the context of their own communities (of locality, interest, experience and identity)
- engage and reinforce the abilities and capacities of service users
- support collective working
- bring the strengths of mutual aid and support to bear in the context of collective action for change
- support self- and mutual empowerment.

Community development approaches have frequently emphasised the importance of involvement and empowerment. They are especially helpful where service users and service-user organisations adopt them and have an effective say in how they are used.

They also have a particularly important role to play when the aim is to ensure truly inclusive involvement. Some service users/survivors have little reason to trust requests to 'get involved'. Because of the particular barriers that face them, they may have little reason to respond to such invitations. In 2013, Shaping Our Lives published the results of a four-year government-funded, user-led research project (Beresford, 2013) exploring service user participation and who tends to get excluded. The research identified five key sites of exclusion:

- equality issues – in relation to gender, sexuality, race, class, culture, belief, age, impairment and more
- where people lived – for example, they were homeless, in the penal system, in welfare institutions, refugees and so on

- they communicated differently – they did not speak the prevailing language, or it was not their first language, or they were deaf and used sign language, used Makaton, or were non-verbal, and so forth
- the nature of their impairments – their impairments were seen as too complex or severe for them to be able or to even want to contribute
- they were seen as unwanted voices – they did not necessarily say what authorities wanted to hear, were regarded as problematic or too disruptive and so forth – for example, neurodiverse people and people living with dementia.

A key conclusion of the project was that reaching out to people to build up trust and confidence, rather than expecting them to come to you, was key to challenging such exclusions, and that community development approaches were key to this.

The development of new roles and new approaches

Almost all the roles associated with mental health policy and practice have their origins in medicalised individual approaches to treatment and understanding. This is not a comment on their value or legitimacy. Mental health service users/survivors still most often comment on whether their psychiatrist, social worker or community psychiatric nurse (CPN) is a 'good' or a 'bad' one, according to the nature of the individual worker, rather than according to the inherent function of the role. However, all the occupational and professional roles associated with the mental health system are more or less based on a model of 'mental illness'. This includes social work (despite its commitment to social approaches) and psychology – even if their analysis and interventions are different from those of mainstream psychiatry.

Now, with the advent of self-run services, complementary approaches, schemes for personal support and new approaches to self-management and self-support, it is particularly timely to explore new roles and new approaches to practice and occupational roles. This has already happened in the context of disability, where new roles and services have been pioneered by the disabled people's movement. Here services not conceived in medicalised terms or in terms of rehabilitation or 'care' have developed over the last few years. This has resulted in new approaches to training, as well as distinct new roles, usually based on the recruitment of people with direct experience of disability and impairment. This includes roles concerned with providing personal assistance, social and housing advice, peer advocacy and counselling and assessment. In some cases this has led to certificated training programmes as well as the emergence of recognised new roles.

This has also begun to happen in the field of mental health. It is a development that would benefit from being taken forward by mainstream policymakers and local services, in close association with mental health service users and their organisations, in a much more strategic and systematic way. There are already a number of emerging roles to build on and develop, such as:

- service-user telephone helpline workers
- non-medicalised crisis and safe-house workers
- peer advocates
- peer advice workers
- employment and support workers
- non-medicalised support workers.

But the general crisis in UK mental health policy and provision and the powerful resistance of psychiatric institutions mean that this is not happening to any great extent, or in some cases is being subverted. Such roles need to be explored, education and training developed (and training materials produced) and schemes for accreditation established to create a range of new workers, both alongside and replacing traditional mental health ones. There is also a place for developing new materials and input to support traditional roles (for example, in social work, occupational therapy and nursing) to address and develop Mad Studies and more social approaches to madness and distress and to explore their implications for the development of conventional practice. Neoliberal ideology sits uncomfortably with all this, but we must plan for the future.

Peter Campbell, a founding member of the UK survivor movement whom we met earlier, summed up what a new approach to support for mental health service users could look like and how far it takes us from traditional models:

> What we need in future is support that is truly holistic. What we have now is a rhetorical commitment to holism but support remains restricted and dominated by a medical model approach. We need imaginative support which recognises the full humanity of people in mental distress. In particular, in future we should be seeing less compulsory care, not more. Otherwise, crises will continue to be accompanied by unpleasant events like being picked up by the police and handcuffed into a police van, and restraint and solitary confinement. In these cases, what many people need is a chance to talk through the trauma, not have it ignored. In general terms, whether there will be more therapy available or not, there definitely needs to be more human interaction going on, more talking and listening of a basic kind.
>
> It would be great to see the expertise of people with direct experience more available. This is partly to do with having more peer support workers but is also about ensuring that self-help groups are not squeezed out by professional-dominated support. Finally, the future will not look good for us unless we gain more choice and control over the support we want. These are key requirements. (Personal communication)

In the continuing difficult economic times, with the governmental emphasis on reducing state support, Anne Beales, formerly leader of the user involvement arm of the charity Together, summed up the challenge facing us:

> We need to face up to our fears about spending cuts in the mental health sector, supporting each other in resisting them, while putting into place alternative peer-led support initiatives [services] which could radically change the landscape of mental health provision and even act as a lifeline to our very existence.
>
> At its heart, peer support exists to benefit the individuals who engage with it, through building mutually beneficial

> relationships based on shared experience, trust and empathy. Evidence shows that these relationships provide people with self-help strategies that professionals may not be able to offer or even know about.
>
> Peer support is by its very nature a community activity, and so it helps people break out of social exclusion. It also mirrors the language of the personalisation agenda, as self-directed and personal choice. Peer support also ticks the 'co-production' box as it cannot be done to or for us, and it begins to address our own agenda around what we (service users/survivors) mean by wellbeing.
>
> Whilst we can't avoid the fact that any potential cuts will have a devastating impact on frontline services for people with mental health issues, the service user movement should also recognise the opportunity to mobilise and promote the value of service user involvement as critical as well as cost-effective, because it works. (Personal communication)

These words of advice hold as strongly today as they did when Anne articulated them for the first edition of this book.

Chapter 10
Developing a new vision: Routes to achieving change

> Survivor research is developing a new foundation, just as users and survivors are in other areas, such as mental health policy, practice, education and anti-discrimination. This foundation is planting itself deep and cracking the bedrock of the most fundamental beliefs traditional mental health systems rest upon.
> *Mary O'Hagan (in Sweeney et al., 2009)*

An alternative vision for mental wellbeing and a system of support to go with it won't be achieved overnight. It won't be achieved at all if it is not supported and encouraged. It is not enough to talk about encouraging managers or 'champions' to support change, as tends to happen now. If that is all that happens, service users will be reliant on the particular skills, quality and commitment of the leads in their area, their mental health trust, their hospital and their services. There will be the same concerns about the patchiness of provision, with frequently expressed worries about the 'postcode lottery' facing service users. They will still be in essentially the same system. A radical survivor-led strategy for an alternative mental health system is needed that goes far beyond this. Unlike many of our political masters, we must think long term.

At the heart of this must be 'an engine for change', with a responsibility for advancing this aspiration. Central to this is the contribution of the service user/survivor movement. If we are to build on the commitment for change regularly expressed by government, policymakers, progressive practitioners and service users, then the survivor movement will be the key starting point for it. It is difficult to see where else such a radical impulse will come from. We should also remember that survivors have gained a footing throughout the system now through the jobs they have secured as peer support workers, researchers, educators and sometimes mainstream practitioners.

But the survivor movement won't achieve this in isolation. It would do well to take a leaf out of the related Mad Studies movement. This, as we have seen, has highlighted the importance of building alliances across different new social movements (NSMs). That must be a priority for the future, if mental health system survivors are not to stay isolated and easily ignored and scapegoated. It has begun to happen. One of the few positive results of successive UK governments' continual harassment of disabled people as recipients of welfare benefits has been the development and strengthening of resistance and alliances between different groups of disabled people. This includes people with learning difficulties, people identified as on the 'autistic spectrum' and mental health service users/survivors.

But this needs to be dramatically extended. There is now much talk of neoliberal ideology advantaging the 'one per cent' over the rest of us who make up the remaining 99 per cent. Different NSMs on their own may always only make up a minority, but if we begin to build alliances and solidarity with each other, we can readily become a majority. There has been a tendency for such movements to fight separate battles and engage in uncoordinated struggles. Instead, we need to build trust and experience in developing more equal relations and working alliances with each other. Once we recognise the importance of intersectionality – that there are so many overlaps between us, reflecting the frequent multiplicities of our identities – this becomes an even more realistic and achievable goal. It should be a priority. A first step should also be drawing on the philosophy and theory-building of the Mad Studies movement. That certainly is one of my priorities as a mental health service user/survivor.

Routes to change

A number of key routes to change can be identified, if we are to advance the progressive principles and approaches to support set out in the last two chapters. These include:

- strengthening user-controlled organisations
- self-education and personal prevention
- societal education and prevention
- valuing user experience in the workforce
- continuity of support
- supporting user research and evaluation
- the centrality of service user/survivor knowledges
- developing quality, embracing user-defined standards
- ensuring a reliable and adequate income
- a transformed labour market – inclusive and less stressful.

I will look at each of these in turn in more detail.

Strengthening user-controlled organisations

User-controlled organisations have been the key active expression of survivor and other service user movements. These are organisations controlled by the people they are intended for, rather than by other groups.

Independent, constituted user-controlled organisations have existed for nearly half a century. They have grown in number, effectiveness and influence but, as we have seen more recently, this progress has been stalled by lack of funding and other cuts. Nonetheless local, regional, national, international and global organisations exist. There has been particular progress in the Global North, but developments have also been taking place in the Global South and its low- and middle-income countries.

They are greatly valued by many mental health service users/survivors. It has long been argued by disabled people and other service users that they provide the best route to developing personal empowerment and generating the impetus for progressive reform, both within and beyond the service system. Colin Barnes, Professor of Disability Studies and long-term disability activist, has charted their origins in the disabled people's movement and the continuing uncertainties it has faced in the UK. He says:

> Since the 1970s, grass-roots user-controlled organisations, often referred to as Centres for Independent Living or CILs, have led the struggle for meaningful policies and services with which to eradicate the inequality and exclusion encountered by the overwhelming majority of disabled people, their families and service users generally. In 2000 there were over 80 user-controlled groups operating across the UK providing a range of independent living services with over half delivering direct payment-type support systems to disabled people, their families and other service users. (Personal communication)

Yet, despite government commitments (that were never fulfilled) to ensure that every local authority had a CIL-type organisation by the year 2010, local user-controlled service providers have been closing at an alarming rate. Decades of under-funding and limited resources have meant that both local and national user-controlled agencies are severely disadvantaged in the increasingly competitive market for local and national contracts to provide independent living and direct payment-type services.

Hence access to meaningful local user-led support and direct payments/personal budgets-type schemes is a postcode lottery. All of this is directly at odds with government rhetoric espousing the need for independent living and the realisation of equal opportunities for disabled people and service users.

For mental health service users, user-controlled organisations have long provided a resource both for mutual aid and for positive social development. They play a crucial role in making possible what Judi Chamberlin called 'consciousness-raising', what the Latin American educator Paulo Friere called 'conscientization', what the US black civil rights movement called 'empowerment', and what some UK service user/survivor organisations now call 'capacity-building'. A crucial element of all these ideas is the enhanced ability they make possible to see one's self in a new and positive light and make the political connections with the world in which one lives. This is an ongoing process that enables us better to understand ourselves and the psychiatric system, how it sees and categorises us and how we can challenge this through recognising our potential for change.

Service users have repeatedly called for adequate state funding for such independent organisations. We know that they can generate their own income through providing goods and services, but they need pump-priming with funding and other resources if they are to get off the ground and build their own and service users' capacity. They may also need ongoing core funding until the routine discrimination and exclusion they face is effectively reduced. They will also benefit from ongoing public financial support to develop their own network and infrastructure to help give them coherence, security and a more powerful independent voice.

Through outreach initiatives, they can provide one of the most effective routes to enabling broad and diverse involvement, as well as reaching out to include the views of service users who may not want to get actively involved.

They play a central role in the thinking of service users, for example, providing the essential support and resources to enable the widest range of service users to access direct payments and personal budgets with confidence and without burden. Yet they are still both inadequately and insecurely funded and, as we have seen, this has been getting worse. Frequently they rely on voluntary unpaid effort, without the essential infrastructure to maintain their effective operation, or are dependent on a sole service-user worker, often working part-time and therefore vulnerable to burn-out. As a result, organisations frequently fold. In some areas there isn't such an organisation and service users are put at unacceptable risk.

Bearing in mind the importance attached by government and statutory services to user involvement – at least rhetorically – and the widespread view among service users that user-controlled organisations provide the crucial basis to enable it to happen and flourish, this is a fundamental problem. A strategic and systematic approach to the funding of user-controlled organisations is urgently required at national level. They are the bricks and mortar of the service-user/survivor movement. Secure and adequate funding that enables organisations to plan and develop effectively is essential. Specific support for Black and ethnic minority user-controlled organisations and adequate funding for outreach work with local Black and minority ethnic communities are also essential.

As Colin Barnes makes clear, without such user-controlled organisations, the crucial user-led services and support that we discussed in the last chapter are likely to be marginalised:

> User-controlled services are quite different from traditional top-down provision run and controlled by professionals.
>
> Traditional top-down professionally led services are almost exclusively still organised around individualistic deficit/medical models of disability and disadvantage and delivered by a vast army of professional helpers. The end result is the gradual but inevitable disempowerment of the overwhelming majority of service users and their families.
>
> In contrast, user-controlled services were devised and developed by organisations controlled and run by service users. Today references to these services and the principles upon which they are based permeate almost all government and professionally led rhetoric on 'social care'.
>
> Yet this has not been matched by meaningful policies and funding with which to develop further user-controlled service providers. Over the last decade there has been a significant decline in these organisations. Consequently control of the support systems for the growing numbers of service users remains, and is likely to remain so in the future, with professionally led agencies and large charities; the very opposite of what is needed. (Personal communication)

Self-education and personal prevention

Most of us start by being personally ill-equipped to deal with madness and distress and the responses they tend to generate. Facing madness and distress for the first time is perhaps also the worst time to try to equip yourself to deal with it. Crisis and vulnerability do not make learning easy. When we are frightened, uncertain, confused and disorientated, we can find it very difficult to put into practice the skills and techniques that we use to help negotiate other major difficulties. This was certainly my experience. We may not feel there is a problem, or we may be totally incapacitated by it because of all the terrifying folklore we have unconsciously learned about 'going mad' and being 'mentally ill'. The people around us are likely to be just as frightened and in just as vulnerable a position. It is difficult to overstate the power of the fear of going mad in societies like ours – however rarely such matters may be discussed.

This is why it is important that madness and distress are subjects that we can learn (and talk) about (with reliable, independent information) from our earliest days. There is an important early role here for schools and education services, from primary and pre-school onwards. And we need to be able to do this without being constrained by narrow, traditional, medicalised understandings. Children are expected to learn how to look after themselves physically. The same attention is rarely paid to equipping them to take care of their mental wellbeing, even though childhood and adolescence can be times of particular difficulty.

And it's not just about providing people with helpful learning. Children are bombarded with 'mentalist' imagery. It is important to challenge conventional negative stereotypes of 'mad people' that are as commonplace on children's TV and in comics and kids' magazines as in adult media (sometimes, though, co-existing with really helpful first-hand accounts by children and young people who have experienced distress).

Education about mental wellbeing issues should be a central component in the national curriculum and specifically in citizenship education, from primary school onwards. It should address the whole range of issues, from rights and stigma to support and self-management. This is a process that needs to permeate all aspects of society, opposing the mentalist imagery and assumptions that still predominate. Some television soaps have begun to address issues of disability in a positive, informed and anti-discriminatory and inclusive way, and this is to be welcomed. With some exceptions, the same has yet to happen effectively for mental health issues. There is also an important role here for employers, supporting people with experience as mental health service users to join (and, importantly, stay in) the workforce and spreading the word that they have a contribution to make.

There is now a vast amount of clear, helpful information available about 'mental health' matters, much of it produced by survivors and their allies. But madness and distress are still so much taboo subjects and the dominant (popular as well as professional) discussion about them is so bound up in fear and internalised oppression that it is still hard for many people routinely to turn to them. We all need to be equipped to recognise the early warning signs, to have a better understanding of what might be happening. But this is not a task that should be left to the individual. Just as we are finding out more about diet and alcohol use, sports injuries and preparation for retirement, so more needs to be done at an infrastructural level to equip individuals to be able to recognise, acknowledge and respond to madness, distress and using mental health services as potential aspects of *all* our lives.

Societal education and prevention

Given that madness and distress have important social relations – with the wider world we live in, its culture, attitudes and material realities – it takes more than the individual, their family and friends to make it okay. It takes all of us.

Health promotion and education have so far mainly been framed in individualist terms, aiming to get the individual to adopt more healthy ways of living. Clearly this can be helpful in the context of mental health too, but it is not enough on its own. A broader social approach is also needed that takes account not only of individual experience but also of the effects of social oppressions and barriers on people's mental (as well as physical) wellbeing. This has been made very clear during the pandemic and ensuing lockdowns. We know that disempowerment, discrimination, trauma, oppression and inequality all play their part in engendering distress. As a result, there are particular problems for people at undue risk of facing such oppression, like women and people from the LGBTQIA+ and Black and minority ethnic communities.

We also know that pressures from poor working conditions, poverty and social and family breakdown can all contribute to personal distress and breakdown. To provide the basis for prevention and education at societal levels, it would be helpful to identify the elements that are likely to have damaging effects on people's psychological wellbeing in a more coherent and systematic way; to monitor and audit them and to explore ways of minimising damaging effects. It should be a routine task of social policy to undertake cost-benefit analyses of existing policies and arrangements, as well as pioneer new developments in public policy, and evaluate their implications and likely impact on madness and distress.

The financial costs of madness and distress are massive. Mental health provision is costly, even though services are seriously underfunded and many service users still experience them as negative and of very limited help. Public policy needs to be subjected to broader, more rigorous evaluation that takes account of the human and financial costs generated by the creation and perpetuation of distress. In this way, it would be possible to develop indices that can provide a more helpful basis for informing and interpreting the economics of policy and take account of the frequently neglected psychological costs of market and state policies.

There is also one specific area for priority attention: the negative role that parts of the media play in the construction of madness and distress. Mental health service users identify stigma as one of the fundamental problems they face. Stigma perpetuates hostility, misunderstanding and exclusion. It is time that enforceable and effective codes of conduct were developed in association with service users and implemented to regulate the media's presentation of 'mental health' issues and mental health service users. Mentalist language like 'loony', 'nutter', 'schizo' and the rest need to be challenged, as should the tendency of the tabloid press to 'racialise' issues of violence in relation to mental health service users. This is one specific area for regulation and change that could have a rapid impact on public understanding. It is also likely to help curb the rising levels of hate crime against a range of groups, including disabled people and mental health service users.

In recent years growing attention has been paid to the negative stereotyping and stigma associated with mental health issues. There have been costly, large-scale anti-stigma campaigns, which have tended to focus on 'public education'. It is debatable how much good they can do, as long as politicians, policymakers and the media themselves continue to stereotype and scapegoat mental health service users/survivors as 'benefits scroungers', violent people and malingerers, as we have increasingly seen in recent years. Such powerful opinion-formers, individuals and institutions need to be prioritised as candidates for re-education if madness and distress are truly to come out of the closet and no longer feel like taboo subjects.

Valuing user experience in the workforce

There is still a strongly ambivalent attitude to the experience of using mental health services in health and social care services. Some workers with such lived experience report that, while these are policy areas where greater understanding of such issues might be expected, often their experience has been the opposite and conventional commercial organisations have shown better understanding, more supportive attitudes and responses.

People who have experienced distress while working in the health and social care sectors frequently report negative responses, being sidelined and seen as no longer suitable for promotion, and being encouraged to leave. Some people are reluctant to be open about their experience of distress for fear of discrimination and negative repercussions. We can see why when cuts and worsening workplace conditions have actually increased in recent years. Just one example is the problem of workplace bullying in the NHS, which makes it hard even for staff to speak out about worsening conditions and care.

At the same time, as a result of pioneering initiatives and growing recognition of the importance of paid employment for the self-esteem and wellbeing of mental health service users, increasing efforts are now being made to support the involvement of people with experience as mental health service users in the health care workforce. These have demonstrated the capacity of a wide range of people with such experience to make an effective contribution, which can also have major personal benefits.

If such developments are to expand and mental health workers' experiences of distress are to be more positively addressed, health and social care policy and services must be encouraged to develop a more positive approach to direct experience of mental distress in their workforce. This will not only make it more possible that the most appropriate and supportive response can be made to such experience. It will also make it possible for people with direct experience of distress to make an even greater contribution as service providers – something we know service users value. It is important that this development is systematically taken forward and carefully monitored and evaluated to ensure that people with experience as service users have the same opportunities as other workers, are not ghettoised in lower-status, lower-paid (or narrowly-interpreted 'user involvement') work, have positive career opportunities and that employment opportunities are primarily developed to meet the needs of service-user workers rather than the organisational interests of the service system.

As in other areas of employment, it will mean re-examining employment practices to ensure they are flexible and supportive so that they minimise rather than exacerbate emotional distress and occupational stress. While equalities legislation is not strong in the UK, it does offer some basis for challenging discrimination and improving survivors' experience in employment: for example, through negotiating and agreeing 'reasonable adjustments' under disability discrimination and equalities legislation to enable them to work on more equal terms. However, reductions in access to legal aid have also undermined the value of such legislation.

Continuity of support

The large-scale adoption of a 'mental illness'-based approach to distress has meant that responses have tended to be framed in terms of 'treatment'. Some diagnostic categories have tended to be seen as long lasting, or even permanent and 'incurable'. Generally though, as with physical illness, the assumption is that the purpose of mental health provision is to provide 'treatment' in order that people can 'get better'. This has tended to mean that support is reduced or removed as soon as people's situations are seen to improve, they feel they are more able to do things and they have got over a crisis or 'bad time'.

This is the routine experience of many mental health service users and it is one that they frequently find very unhelpful and destabilising. While getting back into the routine of life, finding a job and having more control over their lives are taken to mean that 'treatment' has 'worked' and is no longer needed, many service users feel that they need support at that point just as much as before (sometimes more). This model of providing support when things are bad and removing it when service users are seen to be 'better' is likely to gain even greater force now with the widespread adoption of a 'recovery' model in the UK, as we discussed in the previous chapter. Although it is officially seen as offering hope, and as positive, this model is firmly based on a 'mental illness' approach to distress and reflects its shortcomings.

As has been said, it is likely to be much more helpful to think of support for mental health service users in similar terms to the way it is understood for other people identified as disabled. Here there is an understanding that what people need is ongoing support, and that, while the nature of that support may change, the need for it may be long-lasting or indeed constant if they are to function fully as equal citizens and enjoy agency and independence to the best of their abilities. Mental health service users may still need support when they are back in work and have their own informal support arrangements in place. This should not be seen as a reason for removing or reducing support or a sign of inherent dependence. This is the equivalent of taking away a disabled person's wheelchair and other mobility or communication aids. Service users' definitions of their support needs should be central to policy and practice and simplistic assumptions based on cost-driven notions of 'recovery' need to be subjected to fundamental review.

Speaking personally, as I have come to know myself better, I have realised that sometimes some situations are more difficult for me to deal with than others, and I try to equip myself accordingly to deal with them. My distress or madness is part of who I am. It might be nice if it went away, but I'm not expecting that any time soon. Of course, we are all different. It is something I have to manage, not ignore nor deny, and hopefully I can manage it with help, without having to turn again to the psychiatric system. Touching wood!!

Supporting user research and evaluation

In just the last few decades, a radical new idea has entered research and evaluation. It now has the formal support of government, many statutory and non-statutory funders, progressive researchers, research organisations – and service users and their organisations. Key new organisations have developed to take the idea forward in health and social care research. It is meant to underpin the work of the government's National Institute for Health and Care Research and all publicly funded research.

This is the idea and practice of service-user involvement in research. The aim is to ensure that the viewpoints of service users are included in the production, development and institutions of research. The goal is to take account of service users' perspectives and understandings, as well as those of other stakeholders. Service users may be involved in all aspects of research projects, from identifying the research focus and question(s), to undertaking research, data collection, collation, analysis and writing up, as well as dissemination and follow-up action. They are also encouraged to contribute to all aspects of research more generally, from commissioning and peer review to setting priorities and developing methods and methodologies (Wallcraft et al., 2009).

There are more and more books, peer-reviewed journal articles and even special issues, book chapters, websites, webinars, conferences and discussions on the subject. Service users and their organisations have not only got involved in mainstream health and social care research, they have also developed their own 'user-controlled', 'survivor-led' and 'emancipatory' research approaches. Such research emphasises a new, more equal process of undertaking research, with more equal relationships between service users and researchers; an emphasis on supporting the empowerment of service users, and research not only to extend knowledge but also to lead to broader social change. A wide range of projects, big and small, is now being carried out in this way, exploring issues, creating new knowledge and making possible broader change in line with service users'/survivors' priorities, rights and needs (Sweeney et al., 2009).

The centrality of service user/survivor knowledges

As we have seen, this issue of user involvement in research and, indeed, the development of user-led research have acted as powerful reminders of the need constantly to be reviewing the nature and purpose of research. Clearly research is concerned with gathering information and creating knowledge, but whose information and whose knowledge – and knowledge and information in whose interests? Much of the research in mental health has been preoccupied with developing drug treatments – reflecting the interests of the big pharmaceutical companies. But as survivors have increasingly said, is this necessarily in their interests? Asking the question, 'Whose knowledge?' also raises the issue of what kind of knowledge. Survivors have asked, are we talking about 'hoovering' (appropriating) our knowledge for their (policymakers') benefit or accessing experiential knowledge for people's own empowerment?

Service users and other marginalised groups and populations have highlighted the importance of such experiential knowledge: that is to say, knowledge that comes directly from their lived experience of the world and the oppressions associated with it. Unfortunately, historically, formal research has placed much more value on knowledge based on experiment, professional judgements and legitimacy. The direct lived experience of people on the receiving end of discrimination and disadvantage has actually been seen to devalue their viewpoints as they are said to be unable to claim to be neutral, objective and distanced from such experience – the traditional values of positivist research. This has come to be called 'epistemic' injustice, or violence, by some academics. I prefer to see it in straightforward terms of discrimination. It adds a further layer of discrimination to the lives and experience of mental health service users/survivors, who are particularly exposed to this, as their judgement and rationality may be called into question, even years after their experience of distress. It is important to give equal value to experiential knowledge, collective as well as individual, gathered through user-led as well as rigorous participatory research.

A growing number of 'user' or 'survivor researchers' are now undertaking research, both quantitative and qualitative, and small-scale and larger projects. As yet only a tiny proportion of health and social care research is commissioned from service users, but their input is beginning to have an impact on knowledge production, policy and practice. User involvement in research and service-user research are helping to provide more relevant and inclusive data and evaluation, which can provide a better knowledge base for policy and practice for mental wellbeing. Both have a key role in monitoring, evaluating and developing more social approaches to distress. They make it possible for knowledge production to be a truly collaborative and inclusive process. But more work needs to be done on supporting and evaluating such research approaches if they are to fulfil this potential.

Developing quality, embracing user-defined standards

For some time now there has been a growing policy emphasis on and ostensible political interest in improving quality in public services. This has extended to health and welfare, including mental health services. Whether it is a genuine commitment or not, over time it has been reflected in the creation of national service frameworks, including one for mental health (DHSC, 1999), which lays down standards and goals for policy and provision, as well as a more general preoccupation with regulation, regulatory bodies, standards, 'targets' and 'quality control'. The emphasis on standards in recent years has been reflected in the development of a wide range of measures, including performance indicators (for agencies and staff) and quality and outcome measures. This has been linked with an increasing concern with audit, review and measurement.

Critics have argued that a preoccupation with measurement does not necessarily lead to an improvement in quality, and indeed may have the opposite effect, leading to increasing bureaucratisation and creating perverse organisational incentives. But there is another issue, which has less often been raised. Such standards and criteria for quality and quality improvement have generally been based on managerial and professional criteria. However, there is evidence to show that what service providers and policymakers think service users want and prioritise does not always reflect the concerns and priorities of service users themselves.

Service user-controlled organisations, like Shaping Our Lives, have sought to explore and develop related ideas of user-defined measures and standards. Here service users identify what they mean by improved quality, priorities and measures of good services. If the aim is to develop support and services that match the preferences of the diverse range of service users, then it is essential that standards and measures also draw on the views of service users and that service users are genuinely included in the process of establishing such measures and making use of them. If the aim is to change the value base of mental health services and move to a (social) model of policy and provision that represents a departure from traditional approaches, then it is especially important for service users and their organisations to be centrally involved in the conceptualisation and development of quality strategies. We cannot truly say that, under current neoliberal political ideology, much progress has been made in this direction, but it must continue to be a central objective of policy and provision.

Ensuring a reliable and adequate income

When I was writing the first edition of this book in 2010, the government had just embarked on another major campaign of 'welfare reform'. Today, as I am writing the revised edition in 2023, further restrictions on welfare benefits have been announced as part of a spring budget. These attacks on people claiming benefits have been a feature of modern UK social policy. It has hit mental health service users/survivors particularly hard. Each time it has mainly been framed in terms of 'waging war on benefit cheats'.

Spearheaded by the media, it has generated a strong populist response, strengthening hostility against people receiving benefits. Even before this campaign, politicians were talking of getting 'a million people off incapacity benefits' in the UK. This has especially targeted mental health service users. That they mostly don't need to use wheelchairs, hearing and other aids and don't have visible impairments and physical health conditions has long meant that their difficulties have not been well understood. They have faced particular problems in securing disability benefits and have tended to be the first to have them withdrawn. Medical testing has also become increasingly harsh, subjecting mental health service users/survivors to more frequent and more intimidating checks and reviews.

What's interesting is that, although benefits fraud, by the government's own calculations, is very rare (much less than one per cent of payments), a huge amount of heat is generated by the topic, and strenuous, sometimes harsh and cruel efforts are made to reduce it. Tax evasion and avoidance cost the exchequer far more, yet receive much less attention and much less is done to stop them.

Levels of fear and anxiety have been raised and survivors' fears that some people might be driven to end their own life as a result seem, in some publicly reported and documented cases, to have been justified.

What is needed is a reliable and flexible benefits system to ensure that mental health service users receive a secure and adequate income. Arrangements must take account of fluctuations in people's situation and state of health, so they can move in and out of employment without disadvantage, if paid work is an option for them. There has long been discussion of the 'benefits trap' or 'poverty trap', when people are fearful of coming off benefits because they cannot earn as much in employment. This problem needs to be recognised as being about the high cost of housing and low wages that mental health service users can expect to be able to earn because of the discrimination they face, as well as the difficulties that may be created by their distress – it is not about low motivation among service users.

These larger social problems will need to be resolved to overcome these difficulties and in the long term this will require a more flexible, inclusive and socially responsible employment market, as well as adequate levels of benefits that enable people to live in decent housing and afford to eat and keep warm. What is also crucial is a benefits system based on a model like that of independent living developed by the disabled people's movement. Instead of framing people's problems and need for financial support within a model of deficit and inadequacy – which then leads to the kind of close surveillance and control we have increasingly been seeing – its aim needs to be to support them to do all that they might be capable of – a much more enabling and empowering approach.

A transformed labour market – inclusive and less stressful

Work is important in all our lives. Paid work gives many people a sense of purpose and a feeling that they are contributing to society. It's also a place where they can have some everyday social interaction, make friends and form relationships and constructively occupy much of their time.

The statistics show that people who are long-term users of mental health services are much less likely to be in employment than other people and that they are likely to be concentrated in lower-paid, less desirable, poorer-quality jobs. They are not valued as members of the labour market and are seen as being unreliable and having less to offer it. This adds to problems of poverty and social isolation.

Getting a job is frequently seen as the solution to the problem, particularly by government ministers and policymakers, who express concern about a 'dependency culture' and want to cut public spending on health and welfare benefits. But, while employment is presented as a panacea for all, including mental health service users/survivors, it actually raises a whole set of its own problems, particularly given the direction that it has taken in recent years, with increasing economic globalisation and job insecurity.

Old arrangements of 'jobs for life', secure and adequate occupational pensions and improved working conditions resulting from many years of collective struggle have been replaced for many – and especially those on the lowest incomes – by insecure employment, deferred retirement, lack of adequate pensions schemes, uncertainty about the future and poorer (if any) 'terms and conditions' of work. By almost all such criteria, things have got worse for most people on the lowest incomes in the labour market over the past decade. The evidence shows that economic inequality has greatly increased in the UK, as elsewhere, and social mobility has been significantly reduced. People generally are working longer hours; many have to have more than one job to make ends meet or to work long hours of overtime. There have been growing concerns about the 'work/life balance' – people having to spend more time at work and/or commuting to work, with less time for their family, friends and children. Despite the introduction of a national minimum wage, pay rates have been driven down as employers seek to reduce costs, and more and more people have had to be subsidised by state benefits and tax rebates and credits when in work.

Thus, while mental health service users/survivors can expect to be under increasing pressure to get a job, the kind of work and wages available to them are likely to add to problems of distress and insecurity, not resolve them. The instrumental nature of employment and the labour market means that both are increasingly seen as major sources of mental health problems in our society. They play an ambiguous role, generating psychological problems of distress as much as countering them.

If employment is truly to serve a positive purpose for mental health service users/survivors, then its antisocial elements must be challenged. It will need to become less discriminatory and more flexible to accommodate people's mental health care and support needs and maximise their potential contribution. Service users will need more support to access meaningful training and education that is geared to giving them meaningful qualifications and improving their employment skills and prospects. At the same time, worthwhile alternatives need to be available for service users for whom even more flexible formal employment continues to be too difficult.

Survivors and their organisations have long argued that people's value should not be judged solely in terms of their capacity to undertake paid work – especially in the current labour market. They have highlighted other contributions they can and should be supported to make – to their communities, as family members, as volunteers and as active and participating citizens. However, too often, the preoccupation with paid employment creates barriers to their being able to fulfil these valued roles, rather than helping them achieve fulfilment and build on their skills and potential. All this is especially important in a world where the nature of work is likely to be transformed by the widespread advent of artificial intelligence.

Postscript
A broader view and next steps

> We must not let ourselves be reduced to arbitrary constructions… we must not let someone else tell our stories and have control over who we become.
> *Sherry Mead (2010)*

At the beginning of this book, I said that fear was a key word for me in my experience of madness, distress and the service systems I came to encounter. But there's also one other word that keeps recurring for me. That word is 'isolation'. It takes many expressions. People experiencing mental health problems frequently become isolated. There is talk of 'social isolation', 'social exclusion', 'loneliness' and 'loners'. Psychiatric services have their own significant isolating effects, because of the stigma and stereotyping that go with them, which of themselves exacerbate social exclusion.

There is also a further irony. There has never been so much emphasis on communicating as now. We have unprecedented means of communicating through the internet and through our computers, smart phones, social networking and media. Yet at the same time, in the Global North at least, there is more and more talk of loneliness and fragmentation. We can also see how the politics that have now dominated the world for half a century, based on the ideology of neoliberalism, encourage division, putting one group, one community, one nation, one bloc in competition with and fearful of another. In the UK we have seen such politics pollute and pervert our relations with each other, as groups like people on benefits, asylum seekers, refugees, Gypsies and travellers are stigmatised and 'othered' in mainstream political, policy and media discussions. All of these put us at odds with each other, and sometimes even with and within ourselves. All this adds to our sense of isolation and the atomised social reality around us.

There is also another key sense in which this word 'isolation' is important. There is a strong tendency for madness, distress and mental health service users/survivors to be considered and talked about in isolation, as if they were a separate problem and a separate group of people. 'Experts' often put narrow boundaries around this field of discussion, treating it as a specialist focus of professional or research concern. Yet, while we know that different things affect people in different ways and that not everyone seems to run the same risk of entering the psychiatric system, there is no doubt that there are real links between what happens to people in their wider world and madness and distress. Madness and distress are directly linked with and can only truly be understood in terms of our relations with our worlds.

Challenging a maddening world

As sociologists have long told us (but many psychiatrists still seem to find difficult to understand), life is largely about the interactions between individuals and the wider world they inhabit. We may not know what the balance is between 'nature' and 'nurture' – between our individual make-up and what happens to us – in shaping the person we become, but as John Donne said centuries ago: 'No man is an island.' We are all affected by the society around us, and vice versa. What each of us does has some impact on the world around us. And society has an impact – generally much greater – on each of us. Our stories are essentially about the intersection of our individual biography with history – what happens more widely.

But I want to highlight something else here that is crucially important for all of us and our mental wellbeing. This is the degree to which we live in a 'maddening' world. By this I mean the extent to which societies and the wider world are, or are not, supportive of our mental and physical wellbeing – it is difficult truly to separate the two – or instead create obstacles in the way of them. In my view, we live in a highly maddening world, although of course this is not true equally for everyone. Some people, in some situations, some communities, some countries and some parts of the world, are particularly exposed. Let me say a bit more about what I mean when I talk of a 'maddening world'. While we can expect as mental health service users/survivors to be told off for being 'different', we also often have a sense that we live in a world that is itself inherently irrational and frequently drives people to madness and distress.

While many people will say that what they want most in the world is peace, we continue to live in times of war and conflict. In the years following the closure of the long-stay asylums, mental health service users/survivors came under growing attack for being threatening and dangerous because of an assumed association with homicides. Yet ours is a world that celebrates the military, has exhibitions of its killing machines, and at particular times expects men (and increasingly women) to carry out orders to kill, unless they can offer convincing 'conscientious objections' to doing so.

Such wars are constant and truly on a global scale, between nations, ethnic groups, tribes, ideologies, religions, colonisers and decolonisers and world powers. We are even seeing a major war taking place now in Europe, following Russia's invasion of Ukraine, with heavy casualties reported both among civilians and military personnel. War is an extreme example of the maddening nature of society. While we are generally taught from childhood that to kill is murder, killing for our country has long been made a large-scale exception, associated with honour and virtue. More money is spent on war and weapons globally than anything else. There has only been one year since World War II ended in 1945 when a British soldier has not been killed in fighting. The UK's most successful industry is the arms trade. The manufacture of weapons and their use is one of the greatest, if not the greatest, polluters of the environment, yet we focus instead on campaigns against the use of plastic shopping bags, plastic straws and so on in our battles against climate change and environmental destruction.

Modern war creates many more civilian than military casualties and high among these are psychiatric casualties. War literally drives many people mad. It is also no respecter of age. Children, older people, people of any age are all exposed to its destructive effects.

One feature of recent conflicts has been the use of 'child soldiers', as well as conscripted adults. The madness and distress of war is most often discussed in psychiatrised terms as 'post-traumatic stress disorder' (PTSD). It is difficult to see, however, how a 'normal' human reaction to danger, terror and the prospect of injury and death can be constructed as a 'disorder'. It is interesting to note that the number of UK combatants who took their own life following the Falklands War of the 1980s is now greater than the number who were actually killed in the fighting. Grim statistics about the scale of long-term mental health problems following involvement in conflicts are increasingly emerging, and these take no account of the additional mental suffering endured by others as a result of people's personalities being changed through war and the effects of large-scale impairment, loss and bereavement.

War is just an extreme example of the topsy-turvy nature of our world and its maddening effects. It is also a world where globalisation and the inadequately regulated activities of multinational companies and massive corporations are praised and valued, yet these are closely associated with the most terrible damage to the environment, animal and plant life and the sustainability of the planet. Ours is a society where people are fined for dropping litter and sentenced to prison for not sending their children to school, yet water companies receive nominal fines for pumping raw sewage into rivers and the sea. Only a tiny proportion of women who are raped ever see their rapist convicted, and sentences against rapists and child sexual offenders can be minimal compared with those handed out for robbery, drug offences and even non-violent animal rights protest. Yet we know that sex offences against women and children, for example, can have a devastating and enduring effect on the mental health of those who are victimised and can be the reason why they end up as mental health service users and are at greater than usual risk of taking their own life.

We know that all the following are closely associated with madness and distress:

- insecurity
- powerlessness
- trauma

- oppression and abuse
- discrimination
- exclusion
- material want.

We also know that they continue to be commonplace consequences of the unequal distribution of power, status, value and resources in our world and our society.

Further insights into the relationship between the wider world and the individual are offered by people's widespread reliance on mind-altering drugs. The scale of people's reliance and dependence on both prescription and illegal drugs does raise the question of what it is about the world we live in that leads so many people to do this. The survivor activist Carolyn Anderson comments here on the relationship she sees between sexual abuse in childhood and onset in later life of 'schizophrenia'. At the heart of her comments is the relation between people's distress and their wider experience in society:

> The abuse can take many forms such as sexual abuse, physical abuse, verbal abuse from a sibling, friend or family member or bullying. All children need to be loved and nurtured and if they are deprived of this basic need, the effects can be quite traumatic.
>
> The trauma of long-term abuse seems to stay in the subconscious and it may not surface until years later in the form of mental illness. It may be that stress plays a major part in all of this and that the early trauma, because it has not been dealt with and discussed fully through talking therapy, may affect how a person reacts to stress which then builds up until their brain can no longer cope with it and a person is then pushed into psychosis and then into full-blown schizophrenia.
>
> My belief is based on the many friends and service users I know who suffer from schizophrenia and whose lives have been shattered by its devastating effects. Many of them have become fairly stable and are able to cope with their illness, but for others the nightmare goes on. (Personal communication)

It would of course be wrong to assume that, if the world became a less cruel, abusive and oppressive, more equal and accepting place, this would put an end to madness and distress. There will always be bereavements, failures in love and relationships, disappointments, tragedies and other difficulties overshadowing people's lives and mental states. But it is difficult not to think that, if we lived in a world guided more by concern for people's wellbeing and less by the need to make a profit, then the scale of problems we all face would be reduced.

There have been some shifts in government thinking and policies in recent years that reflect some recognition of these issues. For example, there has been more official talk about people's 'happiness' and suggestions that more than material wellbeing is needed to make such happiness possible. But such discussions always come unstuck because of the lack of agreement there tends to be about what 'happiness' is and whether it can or should be legislated for. Another political approach has been to talk of 'total place', where the aim is for all policies to be linked and directed at maximising local communities' and citizens' wellbeing and cohesion. But while the rhetoric has become more commonplace, the thrust of policy continues to be to cut local amenities, support services and public transport and give an increasing role, under neoliberal ideology, to centralising policies and large commercial organisations driven by profit and competition.

A third example has been government's 'New Horizons: A shared vision for mental health' programme (Department of Health, 2009). This strategy had the aim of improving the 'mental wellbeing of all'. However, mental health service users/survivors expressed concern both that it had not been linked with any necessary wider changes in public policy and that it would divert resources from the inadequate mental health services available for current service users. In the event, it had minimal impact on the continuing crisis and decline in mental health policy and provision.

We should not lose sight of the connections that there may be between people's madness and distress and the nature of the world and society they live in. We must always include the latter in the equation and work for big change as well as for change within ourselves. We must challenge the maddening nature of society and seek to lessen it. This is what Peter Campbell has to say about a 'maddening world':

> A less maddening world would have got rid of all the negative preconceptions about madness. This would be connected to a much wider and more open debate about the true nature of madness in which all sections of society took part on a level playing field. Misconceptions about the violence and threat posed by 'the mad' would go out the window, as would the critically disempowering assumption that the mad have no insight and cannot be trusted to know what their best interests are.
>
> Of course, it would be great to live in a world that was less stressful, where people were less isolated, where we all talked and listened to each other more. That would be a less maddening world. But equally important would be a transformed attitude to difference. Not a denial of difference, for in certain respects the mad are different, but a tolerance of difference and a revaluing that says, 'Yes, we are different but different and equal not different and inferior. Not alien.' If we could reshape madness and people's attitude to the mad in these ways, that might make for a less maddening world. (Personal communication)

So if we are truly to commit ourselves to a less maddening world, we must address both our attitudes towards and our understanding of madness and of the world. This is a project that is both intensely personal and globally political and takes account of the interrelations of the two. It is a massive project, but once we begin to see its significance we can begin to work towards it.

Developing a true global challenge to division

However, we must also remember that it is a divided and dividing world as well as maddening one. We cannot helpfully address our own experience and misrepresentation as survivors without looking at the broader human and global context.

Three big global divisions have increasingly come to be recognised, even if inadequately acted on in recent years. One of these is the division between the Global North and Global

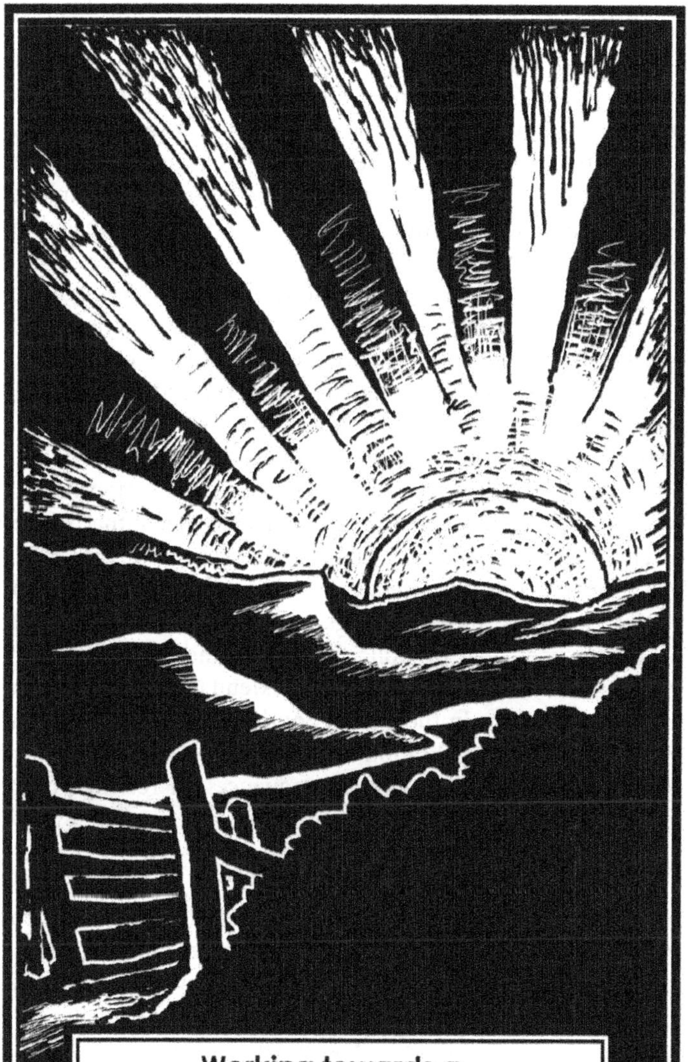

Working towards a less maddening world.

South; the second between colonising and colonised nations and cultures, and the third between settler peoples and indigenous people. All these are interrelated and all are linked with inequality, disadvantage, distress and madness. Thus, historically, imperialistic nations in the Global North sought to colonise peoples, tribes, communities and nations in the Global South, where there is still a concentration of poverty, inequality and disempowerment as a result. Indigenous peoples in many such countries were exploited, dispossessed and subordinated, and some were decimated and enslaved by colonising nations.

These developments are not a thing of the past, although some would like to pretend that they are. Their many consequences reverberate widely. Not only have they had massive consequences on the psyches of the exploited and oppressed – and indeed continue to do so – but they have also perpetuated damaging attitudes and assumptions in settler nations.

More specifically, in some societies the imposition of Western understandings and institutions has meant that Western psychiatric systems and their failed approach to addressing mental wellbeing have been imposed, sometimes at the expense of helpful local, indigenous understandings and responses. Even now this is being perpetuated by policies like 'the movement for global mental health', whose aim has been to extend the reach of Western psychiatric systems in the Global South. All this has taken place in the context of globalisation and dominant neoliberal ideology, which have similar damaging consequences, increasing poverty, inequality, distress and disease.

The part to be played by Mad Studies

So far, the most coherent critique of this situation has come from Mad Studies, the new social movement that rejects a medicalised individual approach to our psychological wellbeing. It also highlights that what is needed especially internationally is an approach to Mad Studies that goes far beyond anti-psychiatry: one that is not only demedicalised but revalues indigenous understandings of madness and distress and seeks to learn from them rather than impose itself on them. If, as I believe we should, we seek to develop Mad Studies to counter the dominance of damaging and distorted understandings of our mental wellbeing, we must make sure that it reduces rather than adds to divisions. One way in which we can do this is by ensuring that Mad Studies is something that challenges rather than reinforces the dominance of the Global North over the Global South. Certainly, psychiatry and its associated institutions have played their part in contributing to this exploitative history and it is essential that any challenge to them does not do the same. We should remember that psychiatry emerged as part of the Western scientific revolution known as the 'Enlightenment' in the 18th century and operated internationally as part of this expansionist and colonialist force.

Those of us who see Mad Studies as having the potential to challenge such failed responses to madness and distress must make sure, however, that we do not fall into the same traps. This has several crucial implications. First, we must seek to avoid the error of again seeking to impose Western understandings and supposed solutions through Mad Studies; of taking on trust the scientism that has dominated psychiatry from its origins; of dismissing indigenous approaches to madness and distress or of seeing them through rose tinted glasses. Second, we must see Mad Studies as a global force that builds on, includes and supports indigenous understandings and responses to madness and distress. Certainly, its key values and principles are consistent with this, for example:

- valuing madness and distress and the people affected by it
- seeking to understand madness in a holistic way
- valuing lived experience
- making the connections with broader material, spiritual, social and political phenomena
- understanding madness as part of the broader human condition
- rejecting medicalised individualism
- not being narrowly focused on and oppositional to the psychiatric system and its 'mental illness' model.

We can see on this basis how it can be consistent with and supportive of understandings like the African Ubuntu philosophy – 'I am because we are'. All this will demand a willingness to challenge the potential exclusions already identified in relation to Mad Studies and to work to decolonise its curriculum. There is already a growing interest in doing this (Beresford & Rose, 2023).

Both the political and the personal

Madness and distress truly are issues that demand that we address the broadest structural concerns and the most intimate aspects of our individual selves. They require that we take account of and seek to reunite the political and the personal. We must also keep the person and the particular individual in the front of our thinking. In our efforts to bring about positive change in line with people's rights and self-defined needs, we should always be reflecting on our own understandings – what our experience has been, what we have found helpful and what we have valued from others. Of course, we must also avoid making assumptions from our own experience that it is the same for other people. This is one of the biggest lessons I have learned in my own life.

What have I learned from my own experience of madness and distress? It is a question I frequently ask myself, as many others may ask the same of themselves. I have learned that, to some extent at least, I can cope. There is much to cope with in this life and world. I rely on the support of others. I have been fortunate to have it. I have good and bad times. Sometimes I feel I have achieved something in my life. At others, I don't. I don't assume I will always be okay. We all have our ups and downs – and I am not talking in some psychiatric sense that has compartmentalised some people as 'bipolar' or 'manic depressive'. Many of us call ourselves survivors. But truly you only know if you have survived when you have come to the appointed end of your journey. I have known a number of mental health service users/survivors who have felt that they had to end their life. But I feel all of them achieved a lot and that their struggles were worthwhile.

I have learned some basic lessons that I have found helpful. Others may have their own lists. This is mine:

- One thing at a time.
- Try to live day by day, one step at a time.
- Don't anticipate troubles and problems.

- Try not to take things too personally.
- Give yourself the same advice you'd give others.
- Try not to judge others – this is the basis for all kindness and wisdom.
- Try not to accept others' negative judgements of you.
- Look for the good in others.
- All things pass – including the bad things.
- You can do it, just as others have done it before you.
- Don't feel ground down by your failures. Everyone has them. Don't beat yourself up. Try to learn from them.
- Doing things with others is the best way – it's often the way we can achieve the most.
- Together, even if on a modest scale, we can make a difference; we can make things better.
- By understanding ourselves better, we can better understand the world.
- By understanding ourselves better, we are better placed to change the world.

I've also learned some lessons from my experience in the psychiatric and benefits system:

- We are all different.
- Our experience of madness and distress can be very different. Things I have dreaded, for example, others seem to have no problem with, and vice versa. But we all face similar barriers and difficulties.
- No one is less than me. I am not less than them.
- Whatever anybody else thinks of me, I have a right to hold to who and what I think I am.
- Madness and distress take many forms. Experiencing any of them generally makes it more possible to understand that of someone else.
- We can get real help and support from others. But the people we can feel closest too and who offer the most natural

understanding and mutual aid are people who have 'been there' like us.

To make progress, we will need to understand ourselves. We will be helped to do that through working with others, and in turn that greater self-understanding will strengthen what we can do together. We will need to form alliances, particularly with other people and groups who face discrimination and oppression. It doesn't have to be for the same reason. This is where our strength and potential lie. We cannot over-estimate the value of building equal alliances with others. Our experience may be different, but the oppression and marginalisation are probably the same.

We will need to develop ways of working that include people facing some of the biggest personal and social barriers – people who find it difficult to leave their homes, difficult to communicate and to be with others. Since our way of making change is from the bottom up and begins with working for change within ourselves, we will always be able to make progress. There is no limit to where that may take us. Wherever we get to, we can have real confidence that we will know ourselves and others better, and feel better about both than we would ever otherwise have done. There is a better place and we have a key part to play in achieving it. Just remember how much has changed for the good in recent years, as well as what has changed for the bad! Together we can make a difference. Together we can make real change.

Contacts and resources

This is a short list of useful user-led and controlled organisations in the UK and Europe. It is not a complete list. Sadly, a number of the user-led organisations listed in the first edition of this book are no longer with us. There are numerous other local projects, organisations and sources of information. But hopefully these listed here can point you in more directions.

Most of these organisations and groups do not have the resources to respond to individual requests for advice and support regarding treatment.

British Deaf Association: https://bda.org.uk

European Network of (ex-)Users and Survivors of Psychiatry:
http://www.enusp.org/

Hearing Voices Network: http://www.hearing-voices.org
Email: info@hearing-voices.org

Inclusion London: supporting Deaf and Disabled people in London
https://www.inclusionlondon.org.uk

Intervoice – An international group for voice hearers:
http://www.intervoiceonline.org

Mad Freedom International (MFI), supporting Mad Pride:
https://mindfreedom.org/about-mfi/mfi-faq/alt/mad

Mind: http://www.mind.org.uk
Infoline: 0300 123 3393

National Survivor User Network: http://www.nsun.org.uk

Shaping Our Lives: https://shapingourlives.org.uk

Social Perspectives Network: http://www.spn.org.uk

Survivor Researcher Network: https://survivorresearcher.net

Survivors History Group: http://studymore.org.uk/mpu.htm

World Network of Users and Survivors of Psychiatry:
https://www.internationaldisabilityalliance.org/WNUSP

References

American Psychiatric Association. (2013). *Diagnostic and statistical manual of mental disorders* (5th ed.) (DSM-5). American Psychiatric Association.

Bansal, N., Karlsen, S., Sashidharan, S.P., Cohen, R., Chew-Graham, C.A. & Malpass, A. (2022). Understanding ethnic inequalities in mental healthcare in the UK: A meta-ethnography. *PLoS Medicine, 19*(12): e1004139. doi: 10.1371/journal.pmed.1004139

Barnes, C. & Mercer, G. (2006). *Independent futures: Creating user-led disability services in a disabling society*. BASW/Policy Press.

Bent, K.N. & McGilvy, J. (2006). When a partner dies: Lesbian widows. *Issues in Mental Health Nursing, 27*(5), 447–59.

Beresford, P. (2000). *Our voice in our future: Mental health issues*. Shaping Our Lives/National Institute for Social Work.

Beresford, P. (2013). *Beyond the usual suspects: Towards inclusive user involvement*. Shaping Our Lives.

Beresford, P. (2019, January 14). Austerity is denying patients and care service users a voice. *The Guardian*. www.theguardian.com/society/2019/jan/14/austerity-denying-patients-care-service-users-voice

Beresford, P. & Rose, D. (2023). Decolonising global mental health: The role of Mad Studies. *Cambridge Prisms: Global Mental Health, 10*, e30,1–8. https://doi.org/10.1017/gmh.2023.21

Beresford, P. & Russo, J. (2022). *The Routledge international handbook of Mad Studies*. Routledge.

Beresford, P. & Slasberg, C. (2023). *The future of social care: From problem to rights-based sustainable solution*. Edward Elgar.

Beresford, P., Nettle, M. & Perring, R. (2010). *Towards a social model of madness and distress*. Joseph Rowntree Foundation.

Beresford, P., Perring, R., Nettle, M. & Wallcraft, J. (2016). *From mental illness to a social model of madness and distress? Exploring what service users say.* Shaping Our Lives/National Survivor User Network.

Brooks, L. (2022, April 8). Trans people's mental health is at a crisis point in UK, warn experts. *The Guardian.* www.theguardian.com/world/2022/apr/08/trans-people-mental-health-crisis-point-uk-warn-experts

Browne, D. (2009). Black communities, mental health and the criminal justice system. In J. Reynolds, R. Muston, T. Heller, J. Leach, M. McCormick, J. Wallcraft & M. Walsh (Eds.), *Mental health still matters* (pp.167–173). Palgrave Macmillan.

Busfield, J. (2006). Mental disorder and human rights. In L. Morris (Ed.), *Human rights: Sociological perspectives* (pp.209–223). Routledge.

Campbell, D. (2022, March 28). Inquiry investigates deaths of 1,500 mental health patients in Essex. *The Guardian.* www.theguardian.com/society/2022/mar/28/inquiry-investigates-deaths-of-1500-nhs-mental-health-patients-in-essex

Campbell, J. & Oliver, M. (1996). *Disability politics: Understanding our past, changing our future.* Routledge.

Campbell, P. (1996). The history of the user movement in the United Kingdom. In T. Heller, J. Reynolds, R. Gomm, R. Muston & S. Pattison (Eds.), *Mental health matters* (pp.218–225). Macmillan/Open University.

Campbell, P. (2009). The service user/survivor movement. In J. Reynolds, R.Muston, T. Heller, J. Leach, M. McCormick, J. Wallcraft & M. Walsh (Eds.), *Mental health still matters* (pp.46–52). Palgrave Macmillan.

Carvel, J. (2004, February 6). How the death of one black patient treated as a 'lesser being' showed up race bias. *The Guardian.* www.theguardian.com/uk/2004/feb/06/race.politics

Chamberlin, J. (1988). *On our own: Patient-controlled alternatives to the mental health system.* Mind.

Department of Health. (2009). *New horizons: A shared vision for mental health.* Department of Health.

Department of Health and Social Care (DHSC). (1999). *National service framework for mental health.* DHSC.

Disability Rights Commission (DRC). (2006). *Equal treatment: Closing the gap.* Disability Rights Commission.

Dodd, V. (2023, May 28). Met police to stop attending emergency mental health calls. *The Guardian.* www.theguardian.com/uk-news/2023/may/28/met-police-to-stop-attending-emergency-mental-health-calls

Donskoy, A.-L. (2009). Benefit of the doubt. In A. Sweeney, P. Beresford, A. Faulkner, M. Nettle & D. Rose (Eds.), *This is survivor research* (pp.166–167). PCCS Books.

Gallagher, P. (2023, April 2). NHS Mental Health services set to face full public inquiry to force staff to give evidence. *i.* https://inews.co.uk/news/health/nhs-mental-health-services-full-public-inquiry-staff-evidence-2249727

Gomm, R. (2009). Mental health and inequality. In J. Reynolds, R. Muston, T. Heller, J. Leach, M. McCormick, J. Wallcraft & M. Walsh (Eds.), *Mental health still matters* (pp.96–109). Palgrave Macmillan.

Halliday, J. (2022, September 28). NHS mental health hospital staff filmed 'mocking and slapping patients.' *The Guardian.* www.theguardian.com/society/2022/sep/28/nhs-mental-health-hospital-staff-filmed-mocking-and-slapping-patients

Heller, T. & Walsh, M. (2009). Introduction, Part IV. In J. Reynolds, R. Muston, T. Heller, J. Leach, M. McCormick, J. Wallcraft & M. Walsh (Eds.), *Mental health still matters* (pp.271–276). Palgrave/Macmillan.

Hill, A. (2016, July 28). Transgender identity should not be diagnosed as mental disorder says study. *The Guardian.* www.theguardian.com/society/2016/jul/28/transgender-identity-should-not-be-diagnosed-as-mental-disorder-says-study

Howley, D. (2009, February 3). Result of a bipolar endgame should not be a lottery. *The Guardian.* www.theguardian.com/society/2011/feb/03/bipolar-disorder-mental-health

Jordan, T. & Lent, A. (Eds.). (1999). *Storming the millennium: The new politics of change.* Lawrence & Wishart.

King, C. (2022). 'Madness' as a term of division, or rejection. In P. Beresford & J. Russo (Eds.), *The Routledge international handbook of Mad Studies* (pp.351–362). Routledge.

LeFrancois, B.A., Menzies, R. & Reaume, G. (Eds.). (2013). *Mad matters: A critical reader in Canadian Mad Studies.* Canadian Scholars Press.

Lent, A. (2002). *British social movements since 1945: Sex, colour, peace and power.* Palgrave Macmillan.

McFarlane, L. (1998). *Diagnosis: Homophobic – The experiences of lesbians, gay men and bisexuals in mental health services.* PACE.

Mead, S. (2010). Cited in *Advocacy Update: European Network of (ex-)Users and Survivors of Psychiatry, 1*(1), 3.

Mental Health Foundation. (2021). *Black, Asian and minority ethnic (BAME) communities.* Fact sheet. Mental Health Foundation.

Morris, J. (1994). Community care or independent living?. *Critical Social Policy, 14*(40). https://doi.org/10.1177/026101839401404002

Morris, J. (Ed.). (1996). *Encounters with strangers: Feminism and disability.* The Women's Press.

Morris, J. (2004). Community care: A disempowering framework. *Disability & Society, 19*(5), 427–442.

Newbigging, K. & Lowe, J. (2005). *Direct payments and mental health: New directions.* Joseph Rowntree Foundation.

NHS Health Research Authority (2021). Public involvement in a pandemic: Lessons from the UK Covid-19 UK public involvement matching service. www.hra.nhs.uk/planning-and-improving-research/best-practice/public-involvement/public-involvement-pandemic-lessons-uk-covid-19-public-involvement-matching-service

Office for Disability Issues (ODI). (2008). *The Independent Living Strategy: A cross-government strategy about independent living for disabled people.* ODI.

O'Hagan, M. (2022). Reflections on power, knowledge and change. In P. Beresford & J. Russo (Eds.), *The Routledge international handbook of Mad Studies* (pp.30–33). Routledge.

Oliver, M. (1996). *Understanding disability: From theory to practice.* Macmillan.

Oliver, M. & Barnes, C. (1998). *Disabled people and social policy: From exclusion to inclusion.* Longman.

Pilgrim, D. (2008). 'Recovery' and current mental health policy. *Chronic Illness, 4*, 295–304.

Ramon, S. & Williams, J.E. (Eds.) (2005). *Mental health at the crossroads: The promise of the psychosocial approach.* Ashgate.

Read, J. & Sanders, P. (2022). *A straight talking introduction to the causes of mental health problems* (2nd ed.). PCCS Books.

Sayce, L. (2000). *From psychiatric patient to citizen: Overcoming discrimination and social exclusion.* Macmillan.

Shera, W. & Wells, L.M. (Eds.). (1999). *Empowerment practice in social work: Developing richer conceptual foundations.* Canadian Scholars' Press.

Staddon, P. (2005). Labelling out: The personal account of an ex-alcoholic lesbian feminist. In E. Ettorre (Ed.), *Making lesbians visible in the substance use field* (pp.69–78). Haworth Press.

Stonewall. (2018). *LGBT in Britain: Health.* Stonewall.

Sweeney, A. (2009). Mickey Mouse scans? In A. Sweeney, P. Beresford, A. Faulkner, M. Nettle & D. Rose (Eds.), *This is survivor research* (pp.165–166). PCCS Books.

Sweeney, A., Beresford, P,. Faulkner, A., Nettle, M. & Rose, D. (Eds.) (2009). *This is survivor research.* PCCS Books.

Taylor, D. (2023, March 22). Draconian migration bill could leave tens of thousands destitute or locked up. *The Guardian*. www.theguardian.com/world/2023/mar/22/draconian-migration-bill-could-leave-tens-of-thousands-destitute-or-locked-up

Tew, J. (Ed.) (2005). *Social perspectives in mental health: Developing social models to understand and work with mental distress.* Jessica Kingsley.

Thomas, C. (2007). *Sociologies of disability and illness: Contested ideas in disability studies and medical sociology.* Palgrave Macmillan.

Turner-Crowson, J. & Wallcraft, J. (2002). The recovery vision for mental health services and research: A British perspective. *Psychiatric Rehabilitation Journal, 25*(3), 245–254.

Wallcraft, J. & Nettle, M. (2009). History, context and language. In J. Wallcraft, B. Schrank & M. Amering (Eds.), *Handbook of service user involvement in mental health research* (pp.1–11). Wiley-Blackwell.

Wallcraft, J., Read, J. & Sweeney, A. (2003). *On our own terms: Users and survivors of mental health services working together for support and change.* Sainsbury Centre for Mental Health.

Wallcraft, J., Schrank, B. & Amering, M. (Eds.). (2009). *Handbook of service user involvement in mental health research.* Wiley-Blackwell.

Webb, D. (2009). Being a survivor researcher helps me survive. In A. Sweeney, P. Beresford, A. Faulkner, M. Nettle & D. Rose (Eds.), *This is survivor research* (pp.170–171). PCCS Books.

Williams, O., Tembo, D., Ocloo, J., Kaur, G., Hickey, M., Farr, M. & Beresford, P. (Eds.). (2021). *COVID-19 and co-production in health and social care research, policy, and practice, vol. 2.* Policy Press.

Wilson, A. & Beresford, P. (2000). 'Anti-oppressive practice': Emancipation or appropriation? *British Journal of Social Work, 30*, 553–573.

Name index

Subject index